BODY IN TUNE

9 Keys In Quantum Living

Gretchen Johnson

GYROTONIC®, **GYROTONIC**® & Logo and **GYROTONIC EXPANSION SYSTEM**® are registered trademarks of Gyrotonic Sales Corp and are used with their permission.

This book is a work of non-fiction. Any names, characters, places, and incidents either are products of the author's imagination or are used fictitiously. Any resemblance to actual persons, living or dead, events, or locales is entirely coincidental.

Body In Tune reflects the views and personal experience of the author. This book is not intended as a guide to independent self-healing or diagnosis. No medical claim is made as to the effect or outcome of the exercises described in this volume and it is not intended as a substitute for consulting with your physician or other healthcare provider. If expert assistance or counseling is needed, the services of a competent professional should be sought.

Gretchen Johnson
Visit my website at www.bodyintunebook.com
Printed in the United States of America

First Printing: July, 2016

The Raymond Aaron Group

ISBN-978-1-77277-050-6

Contents

I dedicate this book to my clients whose questions prompted me to write this book.

It gives you what you need and takes you back to where you've always been.

TESTIMONIALS

There is a great shift of consciousness and awareness that is moving away from authoritarianism to an individual, inner alignment coupled with the higher vibration of community. "Body In Tune" contains common sense tools and techniques to spur your own capacity for change when you engage yourself at the quantum level of interconnection with all creation. Gretchen, through her book and work with students and clients, adds a voice of encouragement for all of us to be causative to our world minute by minute and second by second.
Hazel Williams Carter, C.Ht. RRT

One of my life's goals has been sharing a common sense approach to health and well-being. As I continue on my creative path, I'm happy to welcome Gretchen and "Body In Tune" as a fellow traveler.
Juliu Horvath, GYROTONIC® Method Creator and Founder

ACKNOWLEDGMENTS

A few people create original ideas and the rest of us help to send them out to a wider body receptive.

I have many people in my life to be thankful for. This long list is a demonstration of the community of thought and lessons I have combined in the creation of this book. Time and time again, these unique and singular people have responded with assistance, kindness, advice, teaching, encouragement and friendship.

Many, many thanks to my formative partners in creative crime: Wesley Balk, Ben Krywosz, Vern Sutton, ASK Theater Projects and Karen Miller.

My profound gratitude to Jane Adam, Erica Alexander, Katrina Alexy, Nicole Bernson, Armand Bytton, James Campbell, Hazel Williams Carter, Jake Friesen, Armen Guzelimian, Don Harrison, Jody Jones, O-Lan Jones, Mu Larsen, Mercedes Leanza, Sandra Leanza, Porche Loettermoser, Leon Martell, Mona May, Brent McMunn, Susan McGinty, Mani Mekler and Paul Baker, KW Miller, Meredith Monk, Marc

Antoine Probst, Diana Rosen, Mark Saltzman, Monica Schober, Barbara Schwarz of **GYROTONIC**® LA, Karen Seeberg, Judith Siirila, Tanda Tashjian, Mike Troop, Peter Van Derick, Michele Cross of Physiorhythmic Institute, Dani Beauchamp and Kristy Moorman of Second Story Pilates, Raymond Aaron and the Raymond Aaron Group, my book architects Jennifer Morepaw, Mike Schryer and Lori Murphy, Andrew Brook, and my family and all my ancestors who struggled and risked so I could be here at this place now.

FOREWORD

Take a vacation from yourself by reading this delightful and fascinating book that will inspire you to believe the unbelievable.

With clarity and grace, Gretchen Johnson has written a thoughtful and inspiring collection of wisdom principles that explains how your mind, working in partnership with your body, your imagination and your emotions, can show you that the extraordinary is possible. She provides clear and concise explanations of the growing intersection of science and spirituality.

You will begin to remove the words "I can't" and "I shouldn't" from your vocabulary and open yourself to a new language of opportunity. These principles are easy to put into practice on a daily basis and will help you bridge the gap between your desire to act, and taking action.

Pick one or try them all to inspire yourself to live with curiosity and see your daily life with fresh eyes and a renewed spirit. Discover how you can use the universe of your own body to explore your inner space.

We are all in it for the long haul, and these keys provide a wellspring of motivation for continuous renewal. After reading this powerful book I recommend it as a must read.

Raymond Aaron
NY Times Best Selling Author

Raymond Aaron is known as Canada's #1 thought leader and success coach and is the author of many bestselling books including "Branding Small Business for Dummies" and "Double Your Income Doing What You Love." He has also co-authored two books in the "Chicken Soup For the Soul" series.

*In physics, a **quantum** (plural: quanta) is the minimum amount of any physical entity involved in an interaction.* Wikipedia

At the quantum level we exist as possibilities and a web of connection and relation to the whole.

INTRODUCTION

What do we know?

In a Newtonian, mechanistic view the body is a machine: something breaks down, it gets fixed, the machine works again. Parts wear out.

Quantum mechanics and quantum field theory began to upend this view at the beginning of the 20th century and as more and more sophisticated measuring instruments are developed, scientists uncover relationships that in a mechanistic worldview should not occur, leading to more and more questions. Some of these questions are, as yet, without clear answers.

We know that all living things are mostly made up of four elements: oxygen, hydrogen, carbon and nitrogen. These elements are made up of atoms and atoms are made up of smaller subatomic particles.

We know that each of these subatomic particles is also a wave. A wave is diffuse and not restricted to one location in space and time. The act of observation brings these subatomic wave particles into material existence. We know these waves exist because we can see and photograph the trails they leave behind in particle accelerators. Absent observation these waves exist as fluctuations of energy and information; probabilities in a field of all possibilities.

We know that at the quantum level, every experiment is influenced by the experimenter, the observer. The act of observation influences what is being observed. The observer is part of the field of interaction and a basic component of what they study. Without an observer the universe would exist only as diffuse waves of energy and vibration. There could be no universe without an observer.

"We cannot observe the world without participating in it."
Valerie Hunt, Professor Emeritus Physiological Science UCLA

We know atoms are not tangible matter, but energy and vibration. Atoms have no physical structure. At the quantum level, matter is not actually solid. We only perceive it as solid. At the quantum level, you and all matter are composed of energy and vibration.

The emerging field of neuroplasticity tells us that our brain is not locked into a fixed state; even as adults, it can adapt and change. The brain is resilient and flexible. It can heal from physical damage and adapt to changing social norms.

We know that our brains can be trained not just in physical performance, but also in mental performance. Just as consistent, daily practice enhances physical function, daily meditation enhances gamma waves associated with higher thinking and brain function as a whole.

Neurons that fire together wire together. Firing neurons connect via synapses. A thought generates an electrical impulse which travels from one neuron to another via a synapse.

"Our brain shapes our thoughts and our thoughts shape our brains." Astrophysicist Brian Koberlein

Any daily activity can create new neural networks. This is why almost any skill can be developed and improved with thoughtful repetition. The more you do an action or think a thought, the more likely a pathway will be created between neurons. This gives new hope to patients with brain damage. With repetition the damaged pathways can be rerouted into new wirings. The brain is designed to create new pathways given enough practice. To think a thought is to practice not only brain chemistry but also body chemistry.

We know about mirror neurons. When you experience an emotion or perform an action, specific neurons fire. When you observe *someone else* performing this same action or even when you imagine this action, many of the same neurons also fire as if you were performing the action yourself. In learning a skill, your brain doesn't discriminate between what is real and what is imagined.

The mirror neuron does not know the difference between it and others. Through mirror neurons you experience the emotional state of others without being aware of it. It's easy to be infected by strong negative emotional states like fear and anger, but love and happiness and joy can be experienced in this manner. As much as 98% of your feelings, thoughts and emotions may not actually belong to you.

Self-observation profoundly affects the way your brain acts. When you are not self-aware you can become a victim of any environment, but with practiced self-awareness you can choose what you will react to and how you will respond.

"People don't come preassembled, but are glued together by life… What's interesting about this formulation is not that nature and nurturing both contribute to who we are, but that they actually speak the same language. They both ultimately

achieve their mental and behavioral effects by shaping the synaptic organization of the brain." ref: Joseph LeDoux (2002, p.3)

What is Quantum Living?

Body Mind Connection And Different Types Of Intelligence

I experience my life in a body. I am not air. I am not thought. I am not emotion. I am all those things in a body. I live my life in a body that is made up of earthly elements: bone, sinew, ligaments, liquids. 96.5% of my body is composed of oxygen, carbon, hydrogen and nitrogen and these elements vibrate with an electrical charge. I share these same four elements with all living things. My body has an electrical charge. My thoughts have an electrical charge. All matter has an electrical charge.

How would you live if you were aware of your own, unique quantum signature?

Whether you are consciously aware of it or not, you vibrate with an electrical charge. Your body is energetically aware. Every thought has consequences for your body because your body's electrical and vibrational energy patterns are affected at the quantum level by the energy produced from your thoughts.

There is no shortcut to happiness or contentment in your life without working on yourself. It's an inside *and* outside job.

No matter how hard I try I cannot separate myself from others. At the subatomic level, whether I want to or not, I am exchanging energy with others and the things around me constantly. Without trying, I sense the energy of any room I enter. I know without being told if someone is happy or sad, angry or tired.

Living at the quantum level is living with awareness of your own energy and that of others so you can stop being a victim of this energy exchange and be proactive instead of reactive. You can consciously choose your actions and your reactions. You can move with the energy and blend with it to truly "go with the flow," be in the flow and direct it, align with it and be in alignment with your life mission and purpose.

You and I process information through many channels as the situation demands. We process information emotionally, we process intellectually, we process physically and we process information energetically. Harmonizing physical intelligence and emotional intelligence with intellectual intelligence is quantum living.

Most of us automatically default to our intellect when we are trying to figure out solutions to problems, deciding if something is safe, figuring out which way to move or how to move but, in fact, if you have the use of your emotional, intellectual and physical intelligence together, you have many more options. You have a body and soul partnership.

As a singer physical comfort is paramount, so I have spent a great deal of time considering these issues, studying them and trying them out in my own body to learn principles that work for me.

Body Listening

For various reasons and in various ways, we are taught from our earliest days to ignore the impulses of our body. We are taught to ignore our hunger or overeat, we are taught to go for the burn, to play through the pain. We exercise too little or too much or do the wrong kinds of exercise. We work at jobs that require long hours of repetitive action. We adhere to schedules that go against our individual body clock and body rhythm. We drink too much, get too little sleep.

Have you ever asked yourself "how does my body do this" when you exercise? Most of us merely imitate what we see without actually feeling how that movement works within our own body. We don't know to even ask that question or that our body can talk back to us and tell us what it needs, give us information about our problems and help with solutions. Instead, we imitate something outside of us without connecting it inside.

Where do I find the joy in this movement? How can I make the connections that make this movement work in my body? Certain types of body work like the **GYROTONIC EXPANSION SYSTEM**® and Feldenkrais method re-educate old outmoded physical behaviors and develop new, healthier ones.

As adults, coordinating truth on all levels, physical, emotional and mental, is essential and not doing so can be dangerous.

Your body constantly gives you helpful signals that you can learn to recognize. You can learn to pay attention to how you are in your body so you recognize if you are comfortable around someone. You know if you need to move away, if life threatening danger is coming, do you need to move, do you need to be more alert? You can move out of the way if another driver is going to change lanes without signaling, cross to the other side of the street, move out of the way when someone isn't looking where they are going, see the crack in the sidewalk.

If you live consciously within your body, you read signals from other people and prepare the appropriate response.

Try this exercise: stand up and lock your knees. Do you feel your hips and lower back tighten? Now clench your fists. What does that do to your neck and jaw? Notice your balance. Are you leaning more in one direction? Now release everything for a moment. Notice the release in your body. Alternate back and forth between tension and release and few times and notice how your body feels as you alternate back and forth. Which state do you prefer?

Try alternating between tension and release a few more times, but now notice the shifts in your emotional state as you shift back and forth. What do you notice about your emotions in your physically tense state? How do you feel after you release?

Body Signals

Disgusted, my acting teacher ended my agony. He said, "I would have understood if you had screamed at him. I would have understood if you had hit him. I would have understood if you had thrown a chair at him. I wouldn't have let you do it, but I would have understood it. What I don't understand is how you could stand there and smile."

All the time he was speaking to me, my smile remained frozen on my face and I was beginning to feel nauseous.

With the teacher, my class traced the exercise from the beginning and for the first time I experienced consciously the point at which the exercise had turned and how everything from that time forward had been a lie and a betrayal of my Knowing. My body had recognized my partner's insult and disrespect and responded to it, but my mind had made nice with it because that is what I had been trained to do since childhood and in the ensuing emotional confusion I went into a brain fog, hence the frozen smile.

It was the beginning of a huge lesson for me, and that night I had the most dreadful nightmare of darkness and void I have ever had. During the next days, childhood memories of specific events where I had been taught – not unkindly – to mistrust what I saw, to disconnect from the truth of what I saw, and to teach my brain to lie to my eyes and body, began to float to the surface.

As an adult, I had continued this training, now absorbed into the very fabric of who I was, ignoring danger signals from my body so I could get along and not cause problems.

How does this denial happen? Children don't filter their observations. They are in learning mode. When a child observes,

"Grandpa's drunk." and the adult, thinking they are being protective, says "no, he's just being funny," the child is taught to deny the truth of what they see. "Daddy's passed out on the couch" answered with another well-intentioned lie, "No, he's just tired."

In a fast food restaurant, I overheard an exchange between a mother and her young child who wanted more ketchup. She told him to go to the counter and ask for more and he said he was afraid. What was her response? "No you're not."

It was a thoughtless response to a genuine emotion and it could have been a teachable moment if the mother had slowed down her own response. Instead, in that moment she taught him not to trust himself and deny what he felt in his body.

Since my own teaching moment I have slowly learned to honor and integrate my emotional intelligence and my physical intelligence. I have trained myself to slow down and check my emotions and physical comfort before I react, especially in charged situations. I have learned to be ruthlessly honest in my checks. Over time I have learned I can trust this way of being and my reliance on these tools has grown as I become more aware of ever more subtle disconnects between my mind and body.

Listen To Your Inner Voice To Connect To Yourself

Listening to your body and connecting to your emotions, not shoving them away, provides you with essential information. They are related and yet, two separate things. Have you ever felt yourself breathing shallowly, felt your anxiety creep in and yet ignored it and pushed it down? If you continue to do that over time, it will take its toll on your body. Remember, all thought has consequences for the body.

Ironically, acknowledging that you are feeling anxious, even in a simple phrase like "I'm feeling anxious, where is it coming from?" and letting an answer float to the surface can begin to create calm. You are beginning a dialogue with a hidden, possibly younger, self who may be unknown to your adult self. Acknowledging "that scared me, I'm afraid to do that, I'm sensing that I'm afraid, what's that about," allows you to connect with what's wrong and be ok with it. You can allow your adult self to parent your frozen in time scared self and bring it forward into the present moment where there is safety.

Hold your hand in front of you and speak aloud to your hand: "I'm here. I'm scared, anxious, angry," whatever comes up. Say it out loud. Listen to your words and let the sound go into your ears. Eventually you will start to hear what you are saying. You may even begin to laugh at yourself. This begins to create a new neural network in your brain.

Don't worry that your feelings will annihilate you. Stay with the feeling and breathe consciously and simply (in through the nose, out through the mouth), remind yourself that you are safe, you survived whatever it is that has been triggered for you. Breath into the numbness and exhale generously until you feel yourself come back online. Don't indulge your anxiety. Be the adult and be compassionate with the part that is experiencing anxiety, but don't let it take over. For a free breathing technique download, visit my website, *BodyInTuneBook.com*.

Breathing in through the nose and exhaling through the mouth, calms anxiety. Breathe in for a count of 4, hold for a count of 8, then exhale for a count of 8. Be the adult. Remind yourself that right now you are safe and keep breathing.

Keep breathing while you ask yourself questions out loud about what you are feeling and allow the answers to float to the surface without judgment. The answers are less important than taking the time to be present and allowing the space to ask questions and begin a conversation with your fear and anxiety. Whatever answers float to the surface are perfect. Speak to your hand so you get your thoughts out of your head. Write them down if it helps. You are consciously developing a relationship with your hidden self and encouraging that self to come forward without judgment. Treat that self the way you would treat a beloved child, friend or pet.

Notice your body. Your physical habits affect your emotions, too. Tense your shoulders. Notice your emotional state. Release your shoulders. Does your emotional state change? Tense your face. Squeeze it, hold it. What does that do to your emotional state? Any change when you release? You can repeat this process throughout your body. Notice all the changes. In tensing and releasing you will discover places that are habitually held. Once you have that awareness you can begin to change your habitual state of being. It's amazing how much emotional tension is unconsciously and habitually held in the body. When you release physical tension and learn to return muscles to a neutral ready state, your emotional state can return to balance also.

If you are feeling anxious, ask "Is there a part of me that will not allow this?" Ask your body not your brain. Ask that part, "What do you need?" and bring in whatever it needs, physically if you can, but in your imagination if you can't. Remember the brain can't tell the difference between real and imagined. Breathe and track what you are feeling in your body. Stay with your breath until you feel your nervous system ease and your anxiety level drop. Don't indulge your anxiety. You are playing two parts here, the hidden part and your strong loving adult.

If/when you are ready, ask "what was scary?" Let the answer float to the surface and stay with your breath and the answer. In time, tell that part that you survived, it is safe now. Give it the facts of what is happening now and stay with it until once again your anxiety drops and your nervous system calms. You can ask that part if it would like to come and live with you in the present. If it does, then update it to your present and put it in your heart. Give it a home in your heart. If it doesn't, then ask what it needs and give that part what it has asked for. Tell it, you will come back and visit and it can stay safe where it is. Maybe someday it will want to join you in the present. Take your time. Don't rush this process. It might take several attempts to awaken trust.

First Person Plural or Your Schizophrenic Within

I am large, I contain multitudes. Walt Whitman

Get comfortable with the fact that you are a schizophrenic within. It's not a big deal. You have multiple personalities with different desires and you can benefit from their interplay.

In "The Inner Game of Tennis," Timothy Gallwey described Self 1 and Self 2. Self 1 is the brain and Self 2 is the body. Self 1 instructs, Self 2 acts. We get into trouble when Self 1 tries to tell Self 2 how to do something the latter already knows how to do. With too many bosses the mind and body get confused and don't know what to do.

I know I have little individual selves that come out to play or won't come out to play: the angry self, the spiritual self, the creative self, a physical self, a scared self, a hurt self. Some of these selves can be stuck back in time, stuck at a particular age. If you take the time and ask questions during moments of stress these different selves can emerge into the daylight and be comforted by your adult self who has survived the traumas which caused them to be stuck.

They are all within you and they are all a part of you. With a body in tune, they can become a conscious part of you. When these stuck parts emerge from their hiding places and are given their voice and their place, their negative grip loosens and you can reclaim more of who you are. You'll find more joy and be more energetic. The more you acknowledge them and give them their space, the less they interfere with your life and the more they contribute and become a source of inspiration and creativity. Be playful with them. Don't judge.

The only thing in your life you cannot change is that which you are not willing to see. Anything you hide and won't look at is creating a limitation for you.

More questions to ask: How do I do that? How does that feel? Where does that discomfort come from?

Ask useful questions instead of judgmental statements: that was bad, sounded awful. Frame questions that help you to achieve your intention. "What would it take to _____." When one of your many selves starts whining or thinking negatively, ask "Is this positive? Is this beneficial? Is this relevant?" These questions bring you back to the present and the more you are able to be in the present moment, the less anxiety you feel and the more causative you can be to your life.

Creating Harmony Within Your First Person Plural

Creating harmony among all these different selves contributes to your well-being. You harmonize by allowing each self, each little voice to have their say without judgment. Your adult self listens with compassion.

Memories are held within the cells of our body long after an episode, especially traumatic, negative memories from our own life and even those of our ancestors. Our cells remember things we have consciously forgotten or never knew about.

Candace Pert, former Chief of the Section of Brain Biochemistry of the Clinical Neuroscience Branch at the National

Institute of Mental Health has said, "The chemicals that are running our body and our brain are the same chemicals that are involved in emotion. And that says to me that . . . we'd better pay more attention to emotions with respect to health. Under the influence of massive amounts of contraction, our cells begin to function inefficiently." When we experience massive contraction, there is usually an incomplete release.

Scientists are beginning to understand more and more how the mechanism works but it is known that long term depression, for instance, alters DNA. If the depression goes unresolved long enough the DNA can be permanently altered and that altered DNA is passed down to any offspring.

Think back to when you had some type of accident: fell out of a tree, fell off a bike, got yelled at, had a car accident. How do you feel now when you remember it? How does your body feel? Notice, the question is in the present tense and your response is in the present but you may feel the way you felt in the past. Anytime you encounter a situation that is even remotely similar, your body can react in the same way. That is a place where some part of you has been frozen in time. It's operating from a past perspective. It's a part that needs to be honored and helped to thaw and move forward into the present time where you survived.

The body can be the problem and it can be its own solution. Trauma held in the body can often be released through body movement and breath work. Slow down, move with attention and feel the motion and any emotion that might arise. Reassure that traumatized part of you that you survived it and you are safe now. You can visit my website, *BodyInTuneBook.com* for a free download of a breathing technique to help you stay present in your body.

Quantum Creativity

Being Creative

Being creative is one of the best ways to get in touch with your emotions. Being creative lights up the sensory body, begins to excite you and can eventually change your whole physical being. It can make you excited to be a part of the world with your whole being. Creative artists open up their lives for examination so the rest of us can understand better who we are. By doing your own creative pursuit you also understand better who you are.

Art and music are their own language. From an evolutionary standpoint, art and music probably preceded language. They are universal languages. If you play an instrument, you can communicate with other musicians anywhere on the planet. Your art can be felt by anyone on the planet. Every creation has a consciousness of its own.

Almost anything can be creative if it excites you. Drawing, painting, writing, music, photography are traditional pursuits, but also gardening, walking, dancing, drumming, meditation, reading, re-arranging your home or hanging pictures, or learning almost any new skill.

The **GYROTONIC EXPANSION SYSTEM**® opens creativity because the supported circular, spiraling movements are like dancing and swimming in the air. Your body opens to new pathways of use. Moving in new ways stimulates new ways of creative thinking.

Approach your creative pursuits with a child's mind. Be the apprentice. Talk back to those inner judges that would suppress you. They're probably not your voice anyway. Stop allowing them to make you smaller, get bigger instead. Challenge those judges with questions you might have asked if you had been allowed to be an impertinent child: "Who cares? I want it to be bad (ugly, stupid, crazy, etc.). I don't really care what you think right now." Filter out or talk back to all the judgments and comparisons you use to figure out if you are "good enough" or "doing the right thing." These filters suppress the awareness of what YOU would like to create in your life. When you get rid of these filters, you can see who YOU are and what YOU want. Don't worry if you haven't got it all figured out. Make the first step and allow yourself to figure it out as you go along. You really will figure it out.

Ask yourself, "What would I like to create today?"

Never let anything artistic get in the way. Cole Porter

Making Music

I came to live out loud. Emil Zola

I don't sing because I'm happy; I'm happy because I sing. –
William James

Making music is my main mode of meditation. It is the way
I commune with my spirit and bring myself in alignment with
soul. Singing makes the soul manifest and gives it a voice and
meaning. Making music was one of the earliest ways to
harmonize with others and harmonize with yourself.

With singing I find ways to allow my emotions free reign.
My body is a physical musical instrument.

Find ways to sing. Play an instrument. Sing in the shower,
sing in a community choir. Allow your emotions to have free
reign and feel how the sound resonates in your body. Vibrations
can heal. Become one with the resonance of your instrument.
Let your emotions out in a simple hum if that's all you can do.

Join a drumming circle and bang away, letting the beat
penetrate your soul. It's no surprise that drumming circles have

come back in a big way. Percussion instruments are among the earliest musical instruments and throughout history are found in an infinite variety of forms and formats.

Learning to sing or play a musical instrument and participating in musical activities, a band or a choir, prepares you for your life. It teaches you to play all the way through to the end of a phrase. You learn to pay attention to the details. Playing an instrument increases your memory capacity. Music is a passionate medium and it takes you to your deepest emotions, supporting you to learn what they are and how they feel.

You learn to work with others and you learn to listen deeply. If you are playing in a group making music with people, you are always communicating back and forth among all the participants and reacting to what they are giving you just as they react to what you give them.

This breath technique is known as Bhramari in Pranayama (control of the breath in yoga) practice:

Bee Breath: Sit comfortably and breathe in through your nose. Then with your index fingers on the cartilage between your cheek and ear hum out your exhalation. Hum at a high pitch, like a buzzing bee. The humming resonance has a calming effect and with eyes closed is even more peaceful. It's a good technique to try when you are angry.

Live out loud.

Listening

Music and rhythm find their way into the secret places of the soul. - *Plato*

Charles Darwin once remarked, "If I had my life to live over again, I would have made a rule to read some poetry and listen to some music at least once every week."

Listen to music deeply. Listen to music not just as background music, but sit down and truly listen, let it move into your body and through your body and into your soul. Consciously let it open the pores of your skin and sink and synchronize with your nervous system. Allow your body to move with it.

Musicians do this all the time although we may not ever speak about it. Choose the music you listen to carefully. Your choice should lighten you, enlighten you, make your soul glow. We know intuitively if music makes us feel happy, relaxed, angry, sad, depressed, holy. Does it soothe you?

Nature communicates music in wonderful ways. Wind has music. Traffic has music. Trees have music. Researchers at Damanhur in Italy have developed a machine which appears to demonstrate plants reacting to energy in their environment. The "Music of the Plants" machine measures energetic fluctuations in the plant. A synthesizer converts these measurements to sound frequency, which is then played through speakers. The device demonstrates the plants' capacity to learn and communicate. As people interact with the plant, it is possible to hear the plant responding to this interaction in the music it creates. The plant and the person appear to make music together.

When you listen to music you like, your brain releases dopamine, the "feel-good" neurotransmitter. It can motivate you and reduce your stress level. If you sing along and/or tap your feet to the beat, even better.

I haven't personally experienced this, but Thomas Hardy said "There's a friendly tie of some sort between music and eating." So you might eat less if you lower the lights and listen to soft music.

How to listen? Listen to genres of music that are unfamiliar to you and open yourself to the full experience. Listen for repetition and variation. Listen to it more than once and try to identify the instruments and textures. Notice rhythms and short melodic sequences. Move with the rhythm. Listen to one voice or one instrument and follow it as far as you can. Listen just to the bass or the treble. Listen to the same piece performed by various artists or orchestras. Above all, listen with your heart.

Dancing

If percussion instruments were probably the first instruments created and singing was likely the earliest communication, dance wasn't far behind. Ritual dance for healing and celebration is a part of human history.

Dancing inspires you to move with and through music and rhythm. Play something and allow the music to inspire all your movement the way a young child responds to music. Dance with your children. Dance can reduce stress and elevate your mood. Jumping up and down in rhythm can soften depression.

Physical creative expression can promote self-awareness and self-esteem just by moving through space. It's good for your health, gets your heart rate up. It increases oxytocin and releases endorphins. High energy dance that includes synchronized movements with others enhances these positive results. You have freedom to express non-verbally. You can express your emotions without the limitation of words.

Because you are using your body only, as opposed to playing an instrument, singing and dancing create a direct physical experience of harmony and rhythm. It's an intimate experience.

If you feel inhibited in going to a club, try folk dancing. There are folk dancing clubs all over the country. You can go alone or with someone. The cost to participate is low and they welcome everyone. You can participate in an astonishing variety of folk dances from around the world. You'll learn new dances and make new friends.

There are places where people go to free dance. Do an internet search for "conscious dance" or "ecstatic dance" or "movement medicine" with the name of your city and find places close to you. You have freedom to move your body in any way you please, not in any proscribed way, but how your body, your *own* body responds to the rhythm and melody. You don't have to do it well. Shake only your arms or legs if that is all you feel moved to do. Listen to the music and let the music do with you what it will. You'll discover wellbeing, inclusion, joy, freedom and inspiration. Inventing your own moves can be an ideal way to stretch and enjoy feeling your increased range of motion. You develop your own personal awareness about body line. Host your own dance night and invite your friends to bring their own playlists.

Dance is as diverse and expressive as any art form can be. It has been said that life itself is a dance and with practice we can move more gracefully as we respond to all the changes that come our way. Even if it is just cranking up the tunes by yourself in the living room, it is important to dance through your life. No matter what you're going through, dancing will make you feel better.

Community

Music, dance or any experience done communally multiplies the energy exponentially. When you sing with a choir, play in a band or orchestra or dance in a group, or participate in any kind of community experience of chanting, meditating, performance attendance, the sum is always greater than its parts.

The individual experience, the solitary experience, is important and can be essential for learning, but being in community, with people, sharing a common experience is powerful. All participants may not come away with the same experience, but your own experience will be all the more powerful because you have engaged in it with others toward the same purpose.

The growing, worldwide movement of Kirtan chanting is a perfect example. Kirtan is a Sanskrit word for praise. It is a call and response form of chanting that is not religious but for participants is deeply spiritual. It's a kind of concert sing along where a single chant can last for more than a half hour. The chanting can quiet the mind and, in the words of one enthusiast, "[It feels like] the cells in my body are deeply paused."

According to a 2013 *Time Magazine* article, singing changes your brain and group singing is the most transformative of all. In the U.S., more than 35 million adults participate in church choirs, community choruses and gospel choirs. Studies show that the benefits of communal singing are cumulative and lasting. It's possible that the heart rates of singers in a choir may synchronize, which is why singing in a group can feel like a meditation. The vibrations produced in singing vibrate your heart and all the cells of your body. You let go and feel your heart connect to a deeper place of belonging.

You don't even have to be a good singer. As John Wesley wrote, "Sing lustily and with good courage.... Be no more afraid of your voice now, nor more ashamed of its being heard..."

Some wonderful people join bands, orchestras and choirs. I have developed and maintained lifelong friendships with my musical colleagues. Even short term friendships have more meaning because of our depth of interaction.

With entertainment technology so readily available in our homes, it's easy to become isolated. We can be isolated even within a group of people. Joining a community of people with similar goals is a way of joining with your own soul. Join your soul and join your energy to the energy and soul of others. You'll know you are with the right people if when you check in with yourself, you feel lighter, more energetic. Within the context of community you have an opportunity to discover your gifts and talents and give them voice to a readymade audience. You interact with others who share your interest.

Attend Live Performances

One year I attended a performance of Wagner's "Tristan und Isolde" at Bayreuth. At the time I wasn't a big Wagner fan, but Bayreuth is special and the theater is unique. During the long second act duet, parts of my body began to dissolve and not just from the heat. My connection to the music and drama was so complete, I simply began to dissolve. There was not a sound from the audience in the theater, no coughing, no breathing, nothing. The entire audience was silent and riveted to the onstage performance.

As a performer one of the things I know absolutely is that it is essential to have an audience for the work you do because it completes all the preparation you have done. A performance is not a performance without an audience. The audience completes the circle of giving and receiving. The performer and the audience participate in a continuous loop of giving and receiving.

What I do on stage and my interaction with my accompanist creates an exchange of energy between us and when we have an audience we widen our circle of exchange to allow the audience reaction to our performance; their reaction shapes our continuing performance. We are all in the performance together, having a communal experience, journeying together. We are a community not just for the time we are together but long after, lingering in our memories. In a live performance you experience individually and communally simultaneously.

Humans are social creatures and research shows that we are happier when we are integrated and engaged within a supportive network of relationships. Performances are self-selected community expressions that everyone can enjoy.

Surround yourself with people whose subatomic particles you wouldn't mind sharing. Each person affects every other person and you are constantly spinning off particles and attracting particles spun off from others. It is a continuous, intimate experience and most of us are not aware of it. This affects not only you but everyone on the planet, sentient and non-sentient.

Surround yourself with people whose energy fields you want to share and you automatically feel better about yourself.

Nature in the Quantum Connection

*Once upon a time, I ...dreamt I was a butterfly,
fluttering hither and thither, to all intents and purposes a
butterfly. I was conscious only of following my fancies as a
butterfly, and was unconscious of my individuality as a man.
Suddenly I awoke, and there I lay, myself again. Now I do not
know whether I was then a man dreaming that I was a butterfly,
or whether I am now a butterfly dreaming that I am a man.*
Will Durant

Earthing

Being in nature enhances, connects and develops your
emotional and physical intelligence. Taking a daily walk
surrounded by trees, water, or any other place which soothes,
allows you to create the space to listen and feel your emotions
and feel how your emotions move through your body. At the
subatomic level we are composed of all the same particles as
plants, rocks, insects and animals, working cooperatively within
and sharing everything on a subatomic level. Nothing is truly
solid. To me that means anything can be changed, nothing is
fixed in place.

Shinrin-yoku means taking in the forest atmosphere or forest bathing. The practice was developed in Japan and involves visiting a natural area and walking there in a relaxed way. The practice requires you to deliberately engage with nature using all five senses. Portions of the walks are often done in silence. It is calming, rejuvenating and the restorative benefits promote lower concentrations of cortisol, lower pulse rate, lower blood pressure, more parasympathetic nerve activity and lower sympathetic nerve activity.

This can be practiced at any time by seeking beauty wherever you are and engaging in it fully, reverently and silently.

Earthing can be as simple as walking in your bare feet on the grass or climbing a tree. If you have a safe place where you can do this (probably not a public park where people walk their dogs), take your shoes off, walk through the grass or just stand in the grass or dirt, anything but concrete. Slow your breathing and set your intention to receive energy from the ground. Stand or sit quietly in an attitude of respect and receive. Don't worry if it feels silly or you think you can't feel anything. You may need to try it several times before you recognize what you receive. In time you can also gently gift your own energy into the ground and create a loop of giving and receiving, soothing your nervous system.

You can create a vortex if you breathe into the soles of your feet, feeling into the ground and then breathing with the earth. There is a greeting practice among Polynesians called *"honi"* in which two people greet each other by pressing noses and inhaling at the same time. This represents the exchange of *ha*—the breath of life, and *mana*—spiritual power between two people. That is what happens in your feet when you greet the earth. You are exchanging *ha* and *mana* with the earth though the soles of your feet.

Tree Sitting

Trees and plants have their own energy fields and you can absorb this energy in a positive and revitalizing way for your whole being. Sacred trees with healing powers are found in almost every culture and age. Trees are living beings, an energy form that, more than any other, records within itself the knowledge and history of its surrounding environment. Their cycles of growth, death, rebirth or evergreen are powerfully symbolic.

The Sakyamuni Buddha found his enlightenment sitting under a tree. Although the original Bodhi tree was destroyed, a cutting survived in Sri Lanka. Today saplings from this cutting have been gifted throughout the world.

Although their lore and history was never written down, there is strong evidence that Druids worshipped in groves of trees. The term druid itself possibly derives from the Celtic word for oak.

Taoist Masters observed the tremendous power of trees. Trees strongly root with the Earth, and the more rooted the tree, the higher it can extend to the sky. Trees stand very still.

If you allow it, trees can help you open your energy channels and cultivate calm, presence, and vitality. If you want to try meditating with a tree, follow your intuition. It takes time to cultivate a relationship and each tree is different. Be open and respectful. Feel what is being offered to you and honor it. Establish a ritual approach you adopt each time so both you and the tree can develop a relationship. Visit regularly. You may feel that the tree misses you when you are gone for a longer time than usual.

Put your back against the trunk of a tree or sit in a tree. Touching a tree with one hand and letting the other arm and hand hang free discharges stress. As a source of healing energy, it is best to choose a large, robust tree. While it is not necessary to climb the tree to develop a relationship, it does open up a whole new world. Ask for permission first and then climb gently and carefully so as not to harm the tree. Breathe with the tree. When you sense that a relationship has been established, ask for healing or ask another kind of question or just be in the presence of the tree.

Walking/Hiking

Even when I have lived in the heart of large cities I have always found a place to go to be in nature: a park or a walk a little out of the way of traffic to reconnect to my inner peace and calm my nervous system. Walking and being in nature calms me.

Currently, I am fortunate to have a botanical garden as my backyard. Weather permitting, I walk there as often as I can. On this walk there are small signs that point out natural events happening along the path and the names of various plants. One sign says: *"Roots are powerful. A seed sprouts. As roots grow they move through the smallest fractures and cracks seeking water and nutrients. Eventually they break rocks and boulders."*

The day I first read that I was stopped in my tracks because I recognized it as a metaphor for achieving any task that seems at first to be insurmountable. The smallest step, the smallest force if it is persistently applied can cause great movement beginning with a small crack to a larger fracture and finally a breakthrough of the largest boulder in your way. A favorite quote of mine from environmental artist Andy Goldsworthy saying the same thing is *"[tree] growth is stronger than the stone."*

We've all seen this happening when roots break through a city sidewalk. When a seed grows, all it needs for life is air, sun and water and it only needs enough of these things. What is already there, contained in the seed, begins to emerge. As the seed grows and encounters obstacles in its path, what does it do? Does it overcompensate to obliterate the obstacle or does it go around and patiently work its way through? Does it do this harshly, or gently or softly or insistently? Eventually it finds a way to do the very thing it set out to do, grow on its path.

How do you live an extraordinary life when really you are quite ordinary? How do you live an ordinary life when really you are quite extraordinary? Softly, gently, insistently, eventually you will find the very thing you set out to do and grow on your path.

"Roots are powerful. A seed sprouts. As roots grow they move through the smallest fractures and cracks seeking water and nutrients. Eventually they break rocks and boulders."

Gardening

"We live in a society where we're just maxing ourselves out all the time in terms of paying attention," says Andrea Faber Taylor, Ph.D., a horticulture instructor and researcher in the

Landscape and Human Health Laboratory at the University of Illinois at Urbana-Champaign.

Humans have a finite capacity for the kind of directed attention required by cell phones and email and the like, Taylor says, and when that capacity gets used up we tend to become irritable, error-prone, distractible, and stressed out.

Fortunately this "attention fatigue" appears to be reversible. Following a theory first suggested by University of Michigan researchers in the 1980s, Taylor and other experts have argued that we can replenish ourselves by engaging in "involuntary attention," an effortless form of attention that we use to enjoy nature.

"The breeze blows, things get dew on them, things flower; the sounds, the smells," says Taylor, herself a home gardener. "All of these draw on that form of attention."
Anne Harding, Health.com

Gardening reconnects your body to nature. It's another version of earthing. Gardening fosters a sense of stewardship for the earth. Whether you only have room for a couple of pots or you have a full-fledged garden, all that weeding and pruning has stress reducing effects, in addition to helping you get some exercise. Because it's pleasurable, you're likely to stick with it longer than you would a treadmill.

Green is good for you. When you surround yourself with growing plants, you're getting more than something pretty to look at. The sensory experience stirs mysterious regenerative processes deep in your body and mind. The biologist Edward O. Wilson calls this "biophilia." We're instinctively drawn to connect with other living, growing things to feel part of the web of life.

A study done on patients recovering from abdominal surgery demonstrated that patients with a nature view from their room window healed significantly faster, needed less pain medication, and had fewer complications than the group whose rooms overlooked brick walls. Even looking at pictures of trees and water helped patients to recover faster, reduced anxiety and reduced their need for pain medication. My dentist has eyelevel monitors in each of his treatment rooms showing beautiful photos of nature: animals, birds, trees and mountains. The sound of his drill in my mouth doesn't exactly fade away, but watching the photos on screen certainly eases my discomfort.

The "friendly" soil bacteria Mycobacterium vaccae — common in garden dirt — has been found to alleviate symptoms of psoriasis, allergies and asthma, all of which may stem from an out-of-whack immune system. This particular organism has also been shown to alleviate depression.

Plunge your hands into dirt, water a plant consciously and connect to its life energy. Plants have energy and communicate with us if we can learn to listen. They send out vibrations. Plants and trees make their own music. Caring for and nurturing a garden or a house plant, if you do it in a conscious way, connects and reconnects you with the timeless music of the earth that surrounds us.

Animals

One afternoon I was at home doing nothing in particular when a close friend's dog popped into my head and spoke to me: "I want a dog." This was weird. "You want a dog?" I thought. "Yes," she said. "Katy and Jack (my friends) are so happy together and I want what they have, my own friend. And," she continued, "I want to pick him out." I sent a thought back to her, "Well, that's a little presumptuous of me, but I'll mention it when I see them." And Princess popped back out of my thoughts and I forgot about it for a month or so until Katy told me that she and Jack were getting a new dog. I began laughing and related my story and said Princess wanted to pick out the new dog. I don't think Katy believed me – who would – and Princess got her new friend, but didn't get to make her choice. When I next saw her, I could tell she wasn't especially happy about that!

What a humbling interaction. There is nothing like an animal for teaching you about yourself. Often I have exclaimed "I am a cat in a dog world," while watching my cat or playing with my friend's dog.

Dogs are so simple. They love to get a treat, go for a walk, and having a nice soft bed for snoozing isn't necessary but much appreciated. Dogs teach us gratitude. They are happy about nearly everything, forgive nearly every indignity and love you just the same.

Cats on the other hand don't seem to really care if you love them as long as you feed them. Their subtleties can be hard to read.

I was claimed by a tiny feral kitten some years ago who would meow at me from deep inside the leaves of a century plant outside my window. He loudly meowed and meowed until I reluctantly came out with food to feed him and ultimately he stayed in my care for nearly fifteen years. He never seemed to bond with me. He didn't like to be held, only consented to come inside to be fed or in the most inclement weather and it took some years before he reciprocated cat kisses. Other than food, I assumed he didn't care if I was around or not as long as he was fed.

I had gotten into the habit of sending messages to both my cats (I had an indoor cat also) when I was going to be away on a trip. It seemed to calm my rather high strung indoor cat and so I did it for both of them. This process involved sending pictures to the cat showing me walking down the sidewalk with my suitcase, showing the sun and moon for how many days I would be away, showing a picture of my neighbor who would be feeding them, and then showing me returning with my suitcase. It was a bit tedious and cumbersome, but since it appeared to help, I did it.

When I did this exercise with Jazzman (my outdoor cat) he would squirm to be on his way. This cat was a dude and didn't want no pampering. One weekend I went away for a couple of nights. Since previous experience had suggested that he didn't care if I left, I didn't do the exercise with him. When I returned, I found out otherwise. Jazzman walked up and down the sidewalk outside my window and yelled at me and bawled me out for more than a half hour! His distress at my leaving him without notice was made very clear.

Since I began quieting my own mind and body I have participated in a few interesting interactions with animals. While hiking in the mountains, I encountered a big horn sheep on the trail and stopped, making my body very quiet and my mind quiet and open, sending the big animal gentle energy and receiving his in return. The sheep walked right up to me and I stayed very quiet as we sensed each other's energy. Sadly, someone behind me snapped a photo and the sound broke our moment so who knows how long that interaction might have gone on.

Another time on my garden walk I was sitting on a bench and a road runner stopped a short distance away from me. Again I became very quiet and softened my mind to a receptive state and the bird came closer and closer until it was only a few feet away. We stayed in communion for several minutes before we had both had enough and moved on.

We are inextricably linked with animals in this world we share. As Martin Buber wrote, "An animal's eyes have the power to speak a great language."

Gazing

> *I believe if one always looked at the skies,*
> *one would end up with wings.*
> *Gustav Flaubert*

Looking up at the sky can humble us into silence and in that silence we can listen to our own heart. It is by listening to ourselves that we come to know ourselves. When you contemplate your place in the larger scheme of the starry universe your soul opens to your place in something greater than yourself.

In sky gazing you see and connect to something larger than yourself, even if you don't truly believe something greater exists. Looking up at the sky or opening into the energy flow of the ground removes you from the stimuli and stresses that surround you on a daily basis.

We are all so habituated to these daily and hourly, small and large stimuli and stresses that we only notice them if we create the space to be removed from them. Only then can we once again notice our breath, feel our heart beat and open our spines. We expand our view to a wider view of the world around us, giving us an opportunity to reconnect with the heartbeat of our own body.

Go outside one night and look up into the dark sky. Notice what you see in the sky and what you feel in your body. Notice your breathing and any changes in your breathing pattern. What happens to your thoughts as you continue to look at the sky?

If you grow up with a negative energy space around something you end up perpetuating that energy throughout your life as though that was your reality unless you consciously work to change it. If you do not recognize the stressful and often negative energies that surround you on a daily basis, you become a repeater and spreader of that negative energy in your daily life. By becoming a harmonious body in tune you allow others who interact with you to be a harmonious body in tune. You are causative to the world by allowing, accepting and receiving, not pushing and forcing. Your confidence increases as your connection to your core inner knowing increases. You can receive negative energy from others without worry because you can accept it and deflect it with your inner ninja.

In facing any challenge, try to find a balance between defending yourself and staying in love. When you are presented with a challenge, set your intention to stay in love and acceptance while you take all the necessary action you need to take to meet your challenge.

Gazing up, gazing around, backwards, forwards, above, and below us expands our energy and gives us an opportunity to come back to ourselves and to disconnect from the stress and negative forces that surround us. Open your body to the moon and the stars because, after all, you are made of stardust.

Environment

I hope later she will see and feel a thing about these prairies I have given up talking to others about; a thing that exists here because everything else does not and can be noticed because other things are absent. She seems so depressed sometimes by the monotony and boredom of her city life, I thought maybe in this endless grass and wind she would see a thing that sometimes comes when monotony and boredom are accepted. It's here, but I have no names for it.
Zen and the Art of Motorcycle Maintenance Robert M. Pirsig

Anytime you are out in nature, hopefully sitting in a tree or against a tree, sitting on a bench surrounded by trees and or water, listen for one sound. You can listen to the birds, frogs croaking or the wind moving through the air shaping sound and changing pitch. Listen to nature make music. Even traffic heard this way becomes music. Listening this way calms an overactive, always on alert sympathetic nervous system.

Did you know that even your stomach has a nervous system? It's called the enteric nervous system and is a third branch of the autonomic nervous system. Its job is to transmit and process messages concerning digestion and it has over 100 million neurons, more than the spinal cord. Its nickname is "brain in the gut." We have two brains and they talk to each other. Knowing that, following your gut, trusting your gut, gut feeling, gut reaction, doesn't seem so strange after all.

Geborgenheit. It's an almost untranslatable German word that means so much more than its literal translation. It means the state of having a sense of security and well-being, safe, secure, sheltered, nurtured. It is protection, warmth, closeness, peace, trust, acceptance, and love all at once. It's an awareness of life and the feeling of being alive. I created a gallery wall in my home around this theme. When I look at it, I feel all these things.

We live in a world that can be dehumanizing. Buildings dwarf us and don't acknowledge that they exist to serve us, not the other way around. Our man-made environment should serve us but more often than not it seems that we exist to serve it as we go to jobs every day and drive our daily commute, negotiate obstacles that make up our lives.

More and more we are aware of how our environment affects us physically, mentally and emotionally. Exploring nature's impact on people's mental functioning, social relationships and physical well-being is an emerging field of study. Restorative environments draw inspiration from nature for new thinking in architecture and design.

Create your home environment to feel in alignment with who you are and have it be a place where you feel comfortable in your body. Even if you live in an apartment and are unable to create it completely the way you would like, try to create one area of your home to give you peace within your body. Looking at my *Geborgenheit* gallery wall automatically injects peace into my brain.

What can absolutely make your jaw drop in awe? Knowing and tapping into the thing that makes you feel the rush of wonder reminds you that you are human and not a machine. When you connect with nature you connect with your place in a web of connectivity that serves you, as well as others. It is mutually beneficial.

The Quantum Body - Come Forward With All Your Being

Working with your body in a conscious, cooperative way creates a pathway to the vertical alignment with your soul. It opens the universe inside you and because it is your own discovery, your own knowing, you can use it as a resource and trust it.

The current pain playing out in the world is the result of cultural and individual wounding which remains unhealed. That's why unrest cycles keep repeating. The patterns keep repeating throughout history, different in the particulars but happening for the same reasons. Healing yourself contributes to the healing of world problems. Self-healing comes first by communicating with, and healing, the universe of your own body.

"Hingabe" my teacher said once as I learned a **GYROTONIC®** exercise. My literal understanding of the word was "give back" but it can also mean "yield," a completely foreign concept to me then, mentally and physically, and even just plain wrong. You never achieve anything without pushing and driving yourself, right? I see this incomprehension and

55

recognition again and again in my clients when we first discuss it. As a noun it means "devotion." Applying any one of those meanings to our mental, spiritual and emotional relationship with our bodies is a very alien concept to people who push and push, driving themselves through pain and fatigue because that's all they know how to do, all they've been told to do.

Self-love, compassion and forgiveness are so often just words bandied about with no particular meaning. Truly, how can anyone know love unless you can learn to recognize and feel it for yourself? What is forgiveness if you don't know forgiveness for yourself? You learn forgiveness for yourself and others by consciously working, gently and kindly, with your body, respecting its fears and limitations and asking what it needs. Compassion on a global scale first begins with you.

How do you awaken the body wisdom lying deep within you? How do you come forward united in all of your being? I have been helped by somatic therapies which taught me to listen and take cues from my physical body to develop my emotional awareness and connection.

Constellation/Somatic Work

We are affected by the seven generations that come before us
and affect the seven generations that will follow.
Francesca M. Boring, Shoshone elder.

"DO YOU KNOW WHO I AM?" The scream startled me but the rage was expressed from a deep, righteous place within my soul. It felt exactly right and true. *And it wasn't me screaming it!* I was participating in a constellation workshop and the person screaming wasn't me, didn't even know me, but she was representing me in a field of energy that I had set up – my morphogenetic energy field. She was showing me something true and barely acknowledged within myself.

Family constellation therapy was developed in the 1990's by German psychotherapist, Bert Hellinger, and draws on elements of family systems therapy. Simply explained, it combines epigenetics, morphogenetic fields and somatic work all into one. It is a physical experience which can help heal your brain.

What is epigenetics? The epigene is a complex strand of proteins that wraps each individual gene. The epigene is what turns a gene on or off. Your thoughts and behavior can cause an epigene to change drastically. Epigenetics is an emerging field of biology that studies what actually causes a gene to turn on or off.

What is a morphogenetic field? Morphogenetic defined is "having a specified shape or form." Rupert Sheldrake writes, "I propose that memory is inherent in nature. Most of the so called laws of nature are more like habits. …biological inheritance need not all be coded in the genes…. [e]ach individual inherits a collective memory from past members of the species, and also contributes to the collective memory, affecting other members of the species in the future." In other words, you inherit not only from your family but also from the collective memory of the species. We carry a resonance of the biology and memory of our ancestors.

Unresolved trauma within a family can be carried through generations. Unknowingly you may carry your ancestors' unresolved issues generations later and this has an effect on your health and well-being mentally, emotionally and physically.

An example of a morphogenetic field is running a mile in under four minutes. For years many athletes sought unsuccessfully to run a mile in under four minutes and it was considered a physical impossibility until Roger Bannister succeeded in 1954. After Bannister's successful run, more and more runners broke the four minute mark. It has become the new running standard and since 1954, the mile record has been *lowered* by almost 17 seconds.

Many runners wanted to run a faster mile and together they created an energetic field of potential to run a faster mile. When one runner finally achieved it, his achievement became part of the collective memory—a new energy field—making it easier for others to achieve what was once thought impossible. That is a morphogenetic field.

What is somatic work? Somatic therapy is body-oriented therapy dealing with trauma, large or small, retained in cell memory and works with both the mind and the body. The mind may forget trauma, but the body never does unless there has been a resolution of the trauma. Unresolved trauma stays frozen in your cell memory unless there has been a resolution and subsequent discharge of the energetic residue.

There are many forms: Tension & Trauma Releasing Exercises (TRE), Emotional Freedom Technique (EFT), Eye Movement Desensitization and Reprocessing (EMDR), are only a few methods in this growing field. Their goal is to slowly release emotions overwhelmed and frozen at the time of the original trauma and gently bring them into a physical sensation which can be safely experienced, restoring the responses that were overwhelmed at the time of the initial traumatic event.

Constellation work can be done in a group or even alone once you know what you are doing, and it can be used on any type of issue. You work with an issue that feels stuck and set up a field to connect with your energy within that issue. The energy of the field begins to move your body and create images in your brain. As a participant, your job is to physically allow the response and move as you are directed by the field energy. This information directs your body to move in certain ways. You don't control the field, you follow the information the field is giving you.

A study done using parish registries and harvest records of an isolated town in Sweden shows evidence that a famine at critical times in the lives of the grandparents can affect the life expectancy of the grandchildren. This is the first evidence that an environmental effect can be inherited in humans.

Our generation is so much more mobile than generations of the past. Few of us still live in the cities in which we were born and fewer still know much about the generations beyond our grandparents. In attending family constellation workshops and doing my own work, I have witnessed over and over how unresolved trauma in an earlier generation appears to carry over generation to generation. I have experienced and observed the emotional healing and life reclamation of many as they have healed the trauma not just in their own lives, but also within their family system. The resolution of trauma in the family system brings peace, flow and connection with yourself, generations of your family and something greater than yourself.

> *"As long as our ancestors are still suffering within us, we*
> *cannot be truly happy. If we make a step with awareness ...,*
> *we do this for all the past and future generations.*
> *They all arrive at the same moment we arrive and*
> *we all find peace at the same time."*
> Thich Nhat Hanh

Finding Poetry And Music Within The Body: GYROTONIC EXPANSION SYSTEM®

I became a certified trainer in the **GYROTONIC EXPANSION SYSTEM®**, which I call psychotherapy for the body, because it cultivates a deep connection within your whole body. Its founder, Juliu Horvath, says, "The ultimate aim is to be at home in one's body, to be at one with the nature of oneself, and to experience exercise as a creative and delightful experience." He also says, "I want music in my body and poetry in my body, and I want to be skillful without struggle; it has to come without struggle."

When I took my first **GYROTONIC®** lesson I rediscovered the joy I felt in my body as a child. In my early sessions, my body felt 12 years old again and I laughed through them. I felt graceful and fluid (sometimes). Long constricted and congested areas of my body began to open and come alive again. Over time, the look of my body changed as I increased in suppleness, strength and flexibility. (CAVEAT – this is not a quick fix. It took time and consistent training to make THAT change.) I'm finally singing the music my voice has always wanted to sing better than I've ever sung—EVER.

The **GYROTONIC®** method uses specialized equipment to enable simultaneous lengthening and strengthening of muscles, stimulate circulation, and enhance joint mobility and coordination. The exercise sequences are spiraling, circular movements, which flow together seamlessly in rhythmic repetitions, with corresponding breathing patterns. Each movement flows into the next, allowing the joints to move through a natural range of motion without jarring or compression. These carefully crafted sequences create balance, efficiency, strength and flexibility. (*Adapted from the official website of the* **GYROTONIC EXPANSION SYSTEM®**.)

There are four major principals in the GYROTONIC® method: (1) intention, (2) stabilization through contrast, (3) decompression of the joints and (4) coordination of movement and breath.

Intention - "Intention is the driving force that moves the body." (Juliu Horvath) It is a person's vision that guides his/her movement in the desired direction. **GYROTONIC**® exercises bring what can be unconscious intention into consciousness.

Stabilization through Contrast - The client is assisted to find the balance between extension and lengthening and pulling inward or retracting. This opposition is a continuous wave of reaching out and pulsing in from the center of the body. Each gesture contains within it a counterbalance of opposing forces.

Decompression of the joints - Overly compressed joints cannot move freely. By moving around the joint in a circular manner, joint compression is eased, optimizing the quality and efficiency of most joint movements.

Coordination of movement and breath - Corresponding breath patterns are used for each movement. Generally this involves inhaling when a movement is intended to expand, or open, and exhaling when a movement is intended to contract, or close.

GYROTONIC® classes can be adapted to fit anyone's ability and can be practiced by nearly anyone, including accomplished athletes and dancers, college students, baby boomers, senior citizens, and people with disabilities. It's fun, feels good while you are doing it, and the payoff is immediate. I always look forward to going to my session whether I'm training on my own, working with a trainer or training a client.

I like **GYROTONIC**® exercise because it has helped re-pattern old worn out habits through my own movement. Massage and cranial sacral therapy, chiropractic and acupuncture are wonderful for relieving pain and moving energy, but they didn't undo the habitual movement pattern that got me into the pain program in the first place. If pain is going to go away permanently, you must learn a new way of moving.

During a lifetime injuries and daily use take their toll on your body. The stronger parts of your body (which may be overcompensating for injuries) start to lose strength and the weaker parts weaken more. **GYROTONIC**® exercises help to strengthen and heal the weaker pathways so they can begin again to make their important contribution to your body and the stronger parts won't have to work so hard. It teaches community within the physical structure of the body.

Yoga, Tai Chi and Chi Gong

GYROTONIC® method is often described as yoga with a machine. I first began to explore the body mind connection with yoga. In their purest sense yoga, tai chi and chi gong are moving meditations with many health benefits. What yoga, tai chi, chi gong and **GYROTONIC**® method share is an intention to reverse the flow of your attention from outward to inward. When first beginning a practice find a master teacher who is knowledgeable and understands the body and truly wants to teach.

Yoga is not a competitive sport as is so often practiced in the U.S. today. There are various forms of yoga, but hatha yoga, the physical practice of yoga asanas, is the most widely known. A recent New York Times article highlighted a research study which suggested that yoga benefits bone health in addition to improving posture, balance, coordination, range of motion, strength, gait and mental health.

Depending on the asana, yoga can be a weight-bearing exercise; you support your own body weight in the various positions. The standing postures, for example, redistribute the weight of the body to create a significant weight-bearing challenge. Standing yoga postures also involve balance challenges. You never "hold" a pose in yoga. The challenge is to continually find connection deep within the body. It's a whole body engagement of subtle, deep, continuous movement.

Qigong and tai chi are both ancient Chinese energy practices for connecting with your internal harmonies. Refined over thousands of years, they are practiced around the world for everything from improving health and extending life to enhancing martial arts skills and intuition. These life energy practices reduce stress, balance emotions, increase awareness, boost energy, sharpen the mind, develop internal strength, improve your immune system, or strengthen digestion. They improve muscle function and circulation.

Tai chi is a form of qigong, but they have subtle differences that are not easily explained. The movements are designed to specifically promote the flow of chi, the life force energy within you, and each style generates a specific chi flow in your body. Each practice has a wide range of different movements requiring different kinds of physical coordination.

Both practices increase your breathing capacity. Your body is designed to release 70% of its toxins through breathing. Since your body is 65% oxygen, an intentional practice to increase your breathing capacity helps your habitual breathing to become deeper and last longer, putting more oxygen into your system. My website, *BodyInTuneBook.com* contains a free download of a breathing technique you can easily learn.

Qigong has specific techniques or styles that are effective for specific diseases beyond the scope of tai chi. There are forms or specific qigong exercises to detox or heal specific organs, muscles or parts of the body. Besides being a great whole-body workout, tai chi helps you to reduce and manage pain of all kinds, and to recover more rapidly from trauma.

If you like structure and want to learn a structured sequence of forms, try tai chi. It requires discipline and focus over a period of time. If you don't want to make that kind of time commitment and still want health and wellness benefits, try qigong. With a few classes under your belt you'll have learned something useful and valuable you can continue to practice on your own.

Walking Meditation

"Solvitur ambulando – It is solved by walking."
attributed to St. Augustine of Hippo

Moving and walking meditations develop a relationship with your body. Thich Nhat Hanh describes it as "Going Without Arriving."

Walk consciously by walking a labyrinth or take a daily walk. Pay attention to how your feet move, feel your body and open your mind to your body as you move. This attention opens a communication with your body and helps you to release energetic blockages, negative emotions and churning thoughts. You can embark on a profound and spiritual path through the motion of your body. Walking meditation is a form of meditation in action.

In walking meditation you use the experience of walking as your focus. You keep your eyes open and your awareness involved with the experience of walking. When your body is in motion, it is easier to be aware of it than when you are sitting still. This can make walking meditation an intense experience. You can experience your body intensely, and find intense enjoyment.

The practice of walking meditation easily fits into your life. Even walking from the car into the supermarket can be an opportunity for a minute's walking meditation if you consciously walk the path from your car to the store.

I first learned walking meditation at the Shambala community in Los Angeles. We stood in a circle around the room and began to slowly walk one conscious foot in front of the other in a continuous moving circle around the room. We were instructed to keep our eyes looking slightly downward with a soft focus, to notice our breathing and notice our heel toe movement as our foot contacted the floor. We were to feel our legs as they rose and fell.

Walking meditation can serve as a powerful bridge between a sitting meditation practice and daily life, helping you to be more present, mindful and concentrated in your daily activities. It can reconnect you to simplicity of being and the appreciation that comes from it.

Labyrinths

A labyrinth is a type of walking meditation or path of prayer. The labyrinth has ancient and anonymous origins and is a pattern that is universal to all of humanity. Depictions of labyrinths have been found in many cultures all over the world on pottery, coins, tablets and tiles that date as far back as 5,000 years. Many patterns are based on spirals and circles mirrored in nature. Labyrinths do not necessarily reflect any religion or culture and so appeal to people from all backgrounds and walks of life. The power of the labyrinth comes from the invitation one receives to slow down and go within to a place where science and technology end.

There is a resurgence of interest in labyrinths and it is possible to find a labyrinth to walk in many unexpected places. Many people are constructing labyrinths in their yards. If you would like to try finger walking through a labyrinth, please visit my website, *BodyInTuneBook.com*, for a free download.

There is no one way or one correct way to walk a labyrinth – do what feels right to you. You can set your intention at the beginning of the labyrinth and meditate on it as you walk the circuit. By the time you reach the center you may have had some insight into your intention. You can end your walk when you reach the center or meditate a moment in the center and then walk back out again. You can vary the rhythm of your walk: walk to the tempo of your heart or walk slowly into the center and more rapidly out, or reverse it or keep your pace steady throughout.

Through Movement The Body Re-Patterns

Pain is a result of sustained muscle contraction. Through years of repetition you can become imprisoned by your own engrained habits. Dysfunction in one part of your body can adversely affect other parts, including your organs. The longer you live and repeat stressful movement patterns the more automatic they become. These inefficient and ultimately, stressful, movement patterns can be the result of modeling the poor movement of others, injury, overuse or emotional stress.

Your muscles are designed to work together in synchronistic harmony to produce efficient movement. Injury or overuse interrupts this balance and some muscles become overused while others become underutilized, creating an imbalance which sooner or later becomes pain. Muscles held in chronic contraction will become sore, weak, and exhausted and the excess tension will place pressure on nerves and joints creating asymmetry in the body's postural alignment. As you age, these imbalances cause the strongest, most overworked muscles to weaken and the weaker muscles to weaken even more.

An important solution to pain is releasing chronic muscle contractions by exploring new patterns of movement which can then develop new brain patterns. Pain can exist in the brain when the brain is no longer aware of individual body parts after a lifetime of unconscious movement. Supported, gentle movements performed with awareness and intention allow the brain to perceive shifts in worn out, habitual patterns. Change happens when the brain perceives the differences and parts are reintegrated without struggle and force.

Pain can be a doorway into a more efficient, balanced way of moving. Our capacity for change is only as limited as our willingness to learn. The **GYROTONIC EXPANSION SYSTEM**® supports a wide variety of movement through space and releases strained muscles and energetic stagnations in the body to re-pattern healthy movement. Repatterning through breath and movement, especially the circular and spiraling movement of **GYROTONIC**® exercise, allows your healing to go even deeper.

*"From the word "gyro" (meaning ring, spiral or circle) and "tonic" (to tone or invigorate), the **GYROTONIC®** method is a way of increasing range of motion, coordination, and strength by performing prescribed graceful, circular motions."*
- Juliu Horvath

Training In Partnership With The Body

Training tools are necessary, whether it's an emotional therapy tool or a physical therapy tool that works in community with the body. An important question that should be asked before using any type of training tool is, "how does this work in my body? How does my body feel when I am doing this?" If we ask questions, the body will tell us, "Yes this feels good, no this doesn't feel good. It doesn't feel good because of this. It doesn't feel good right now, but it's moving in the right direction."

Some discomfort in training is not always a bad thing, but you have to distinguish the type of discomfort. Go slowly and with intention. Are you supported in the movement? Are you uncomfortable because you haven't opened this place in a long time? Does the movement feel balanced or are you straining and overworking? Are you afraid of hurting yourself? Can the movement be altered in some way?

Sometimes your brain will want to protect your body by tensing or contracting in an injured or painful area, but your body may be better served by a balanced and supported opening. Differentiating between discomfort that places strain and stress, and discomfort that is temporary because you are opening a long constricted area opens communication with the body and is an important step in learning to respect your body wisdom.

Quantum I AM

I strive and struggle to deliver right the music of my nature.
Elizabeth Barrett Browning

Decisions Made As A Child

"Gretchen, you're at about a 2, can you increase it to 6?" "I feel like my face is breaking!" I said through my clenched jaw.

The technique we had been working on was what Wesley Balk called "facial emotional" and involved showing all types of emotions on our faces, moving facial muscles into extreme expressions, sometimes piling three, four and five conflicting emotions into one expression.

After this particularly grueling (for me) singing acting session, Wes approached me and complimented me on my struggle. *"What?"* I thought. He went on, "I can see the struggle you're having and I want to thank you for trying to do what I'm asking of you." I said, "It's giving me a headache," and then in the face of his compassion, I finally broke apart, "and it makes me terrified!"

I was raised in a stoic Midwestern environment and I was taught that if you can't see it, feel it, taste it or hear it, it doesn't exist. My childhood was disrupted by parental alcoholism and divorce. I learned very early to hide my feelings and put on a happy face or at least a neutral one, a controlled appearance, one not affected by someone yelling at me. I learned that by controlling my emotions I had power and control in my world and it made me feel safe. Showing emotion, as I was being asked to do in the exercise, terrified me because it made me feel weak and vulnerable. I didn't *want* anyone to see what I was feeling. It was dangerous.

So many decisions about how you should behave are made before you are conscious of making any decisions. These decisions govern your entire life. Decisions made as a child can shrink you and your life in many ways.

How many thoughts and decisions you make each day are derived from learning seeded before you had any conscious thought? Up until the age of three you are an absorbent sponge for information and learning. By the age of 2 or 3, you have twice as many synapses in your brain than you will have as an adult. During the first years of your life you discard the unused surplus synapses and strengthen and define the ones you use. The organization of your adult brain is affected by your earliest, pre-conscious, experiences.

Body Intelligence

An important key to harmony within is to uncover and examine any decisions you made as a child. Throughout your life these (now unconscious) early decisions influence you and as you develop and harmonize more and more with your body and emotional intelligence these decisions surface.

In listening to the wisdom of your body and emotional intelligence, allow these unexamined assumptions to surface. There are exercises and practices, like meditation, that facilitate this. How will you know your inner "yes?" Does your body feel expansive, warm? Are you experiencing an energy surge, excitement or are your body and emotions meeting in a "no": contraction, tight breathing, jaw tension, a feeling of enervation? **GYROTONIC®** training and constellation work are great for increasing your sensitivity to your inner "yes" and "no." Question every assumption. Don't take anything you think or feel for granted.

Any time I am doing something that is a habit which no longer serves me, I now recognize a certain feeling in my body. It usually occurs in the same area and as I have tuned into my body, this feeling becomes more and more pronounced so I can no longer ignore it. The feeling is familiar and comfortable and it also now feels restrictive. That is my key to know that I am engaged in an unexamined habit which no longer serves me well.

I joke that "Overdo" is my first, last and middle name. I've always been an over-worker, a pusher, but singing is all about working *with* the body, harmonizing with your body and breath, allowing your breath to do just enough, not too much, but *just enough*, like Goldilocks.

Recently, while practicing a new piece, I was having difficulty releasing my breath during a long phrase to allow my body to take the lead. I consciously knew I could sing the phrase well, but I noticed my brain **would not** release its direction (a Self 1 and Self 2 conflict) and I was pushing, overcompensating at a crucial point. A memory of my six year old self suddenly flashed into my head. I had experienced a big disappointment at that age and my disappointed six year old self decided then that she would always be better than anyone else. That early decision was now governing the adult me.

In a flash I realized my younger self's decision to be better than anyone else had pushed me to overcompensate continuously. My determination to never experience failure and my fear of not being good enough was now *causing* my failure. It was preventing me from doing just enough so my voice could resonate optimally. There was no optimal "go with the flow" because at crucial moments my brain insisted on taking over and making the flow GO WITH IT!

That early decision may have served me well as a child, but now it was no longer useful and in fact, was impeding my full adult experience of life. I have power as an adult and am in control of my decisions and reactions. I can make a different choice.

This is a radical idea: at times I must do just enough, not more, not less.

Question Everything - You Don't Have To Be Like Everyone Else

What is true for me is a big question no one seems to ask much. Learning who you truly are *requires* asking questions. What is true for me in the world, in my relationships, in sex, in career, in family? What is true for me about money? What does happiness mean for me that doesn't seem to be true for others? Taking time to ask these questions and thinking about the answers teaches you much about who you really are and what you think and what you feel, apart from what you have been taught and what was put on you at a time when you were still preverbal. Remember, you absorb most of what you know about the world before your second birthday.

Ask yourself what is right about me? We continually judge ourselves for what we lack, but how about asking yourself what's right about me? What are my strengths, what do I like about me?

I heard recently that for every judgment you make it takes twenty-five other judgments to hold it in place and for every one of those judgments, another twenty-five to hold them in place. That's a lot of work and a very heavy load.

Every no response requires three yeses to neutralize it. A UCLA survey from a few years ago reported that the average one year old child may hear the word "no" more than 400 times a day. Have you ever heard 1200 yeses in one day? It's hard to develop a healthy, intact ego around "no."

Saying or hearing "no" stops the energy flow. Anything said after that is hitting a brick wall.

Asking questions creates space: space for releasing anxiety around a particular issue and space for allowing potential solutions to arise.

How do I do that? How does that feel? Where does that discomfort come from? Useful questions instead of judging ones: that was bad, sounded awful. Frame questions that help you to achieve your intention: What would it take to [fill in the blank]? Speak out loud to reinforce new neural pathways.

Language is powerful. Use it consciously. Instead of functioning from your perceived reality use conscious language to help you function from your infinite being.

Do You Really Believe Everything You Have Been Taught By Your Parents?

Do you really believe what you have been taught by your parents and others? Often they teach you lessons they don't intend to teach you.

I can still remember making some observations that were uncomfortable for my mother and my mother would quickly say, "oh no that's not it." Her intention may have been to protect me (or herself) from something uncomfortable or embarrassing, but what it taught me was that I couldn't believe what I saw with my own eyes. It hindered me for years. As an adult I was adept at seeing something and denying the reality of what I saw and felt. I had no reference for truth because I had been told what I saw wasn't really happening, wasn't really the truth. Consequently I was able to ignore and deny when I was being mistreated, because I had been taught what I felt was happening wasn't really true.

Remember the mother and child in the fast food restaurant? After they sat down with their food, the little boy wanted more ketchup and his mother told him to go up to the counter and ask for more. The child said he was afraid to ask and his mother said "No you're not!" She taught him that his feelings lie and that he was not feeling the right thing.

Mom is the most important authority in his young life and she unintentionally taught him to disbelieve his feelings and disconnect from his body. If mom had said "ok I understand that. Let me help. I can see you if you go to the counter by yourself. Let's practice what you can say to the cashier and I will watch when you go to the counter." If she had taken a couple of extra minutes to practice with her son and teach him how to do something that was still new to him, it would have validated his initial fear, helped him out of his fear so he could move forward. Her attention would have taught him a new skill.

I once took my friend's children to an amusement park. As we were standing in line at the tilt-a-whirl, the little girl, looking at the salmon colored rounded tops of the gondolas, exclaimed in her very loud little girl voice that everyone in the long line could hear, *"GRETCHEN, THEY LOOK JUST LIKE GIANT PENISES!"* Did I deny what her young eyes saw? No. No, I did not. I very calmly and quietly said, "You're right. They do."

What Would You Do And Who Would You Be If No One Judged You?

True humility is not thinking less of yourself, it is thinking of yourself less."— C.S. Lewis

What about the judges in your head? That was another radical concept I learned early on in my singing career. I constantly beat myself up with the voices in my head that said I was dumb, stupid, lazy, incompetent, ungrateful and that I'd never amount to anything. I read a wonderful book, "Soprano On Her Head." In it, the author, Eloise Ristad, suggested you listen to these inner voices, the judges, really listen to what they are saying to you. Is it someone you would want for a friend, someone you would want in your life?

That question pulled me up short because I wanted to be as far away from these voices as I could be. I certainly would not want this person or these people in my life at all. I wouldn't want them anywhere near me. I would walk away from them. And they filled up my head all the time. Then, when I started to actually listen to the sound of these voices instead of just letting them be a constant grumble in my head that I tried to shove aside, I realized with a shock, it was mostly one voice and the voice wasn't even mine. It was the voice of someone else who had repeatedly said those things to me and I had absorbed them as truth.

That was the turning point to shutting down my judges. I could then ask "do I really believe that?" "Am I really that way?" And that answer was almost always a resounding NO! That person told me I was that way, but I'm not, maybe I never was. I am really very different from that.

Do you really believe everything you've been taught, whether it was taught to you by your parents or another influential adult in your early life? Are the things they told you about yourself really true? In your heart, are they really you? As a now conscious, thinking adult, someone who is now in charge of their own life, are the things you were told as a child (good and bad, positive and negative) REALLY who you are? They may not be true, may never have been true.

Positive affirming things can be just as imprisoning as the negative things. It is important to find out for yourself who you really are.

What would you do and who would you be if no one judged you? If you didn't judge you, if those voices in your head didn't judge you, if those early judges didn't judge you? What would you do and who would you be? Listen to your self-talk. What is your self-talk? If you don't like it, talk back to it. Say no it's not true, no, no, no. Then affirm who you truly are. Make a list of all the things that are right about you. Say it out loud. Say it into your hand. Say it out loud into a mirror. Make several lists and put them where you will read them daily until you absorb that list just as surely as you absorbed the false one. Make your new neural pathways.

Forge Your Inner Game

Change your self-talk. Now that you are listening to your judges and you know what they are saying to you and you've made an assessment of what is right about you, what you really think, learn your inner game. Instead of allowing those nasty judges to rattle around in your head, when you become conscious of one say "out Spot!!" and turn it around to one of the things you like about yourself; one of the things you truly in your heart believe. You tell that judge, "No it's not true. You are *[name of person who said those false things]* and they said that, they thought that and put that on me, but I don't believe that. I didn't believe it then and I don't believe it now. It's not true."

You can test yourself to see how much you believe certain self-talk. You and your thoughts are electrically charged and a simple muscle test can help you determine how strong or how weak your response is to a particular question. You must be very clear with your question and be in as neutral state of mind and body as you can muster. You are learning to feel into your body for your truth.

First, test yourself with a simple question. Standing in a comfortable state, spine erect, pelvis, knees and ankles soft, with the soles of your feet opening to the ground (remember grounding?), arms comfortable at your sides, soften your gaze or close your eyes, say "Show me yes." After a few seconds, you will feel your body pushed in a direction, usually forward or backwards. This is your yes position. Take your time with this. Don't rush it or be in a hurry. Wait for your body to push you. You are aligning your physical response with the energy of yes.

Return your physical and mental states to neutral and say "Show me no." Again, you will feel yourself energetically pushed in a (usually) forwards or backwards direction. This is your physical alignment with your no position.

Now test it. Starting in your neutral state, say "my name is *[say your name]*." Do you feel yourself being energetically pushed in one direction or another? In which direction are you pushed? Be patient and remain neutral until you feel your body being moved in a direction.

Test it again. Return to your neutral state, say "my name is *[say a made up name, one not remotely related to you]*." Are you being pushed in another direction? In which direction are you pushed?

When you say your name, you should feel yourself being pushed from your neutral state to your yes position and when you say a name unrelated to you, you should be pushed to your no position.

Muscle testing is tricky because the accuracy of the response depends on beginning from a true neutral state with no investment in the outcome of the answer. It is also dependent on how specific your question is. Your question should be unambiguous and clear.

Information accessed through muscle testing is what is stored in the belief programs of your subconscious mind. Performed with pure intent it accesses your subconscious thinking and what you believe is true. Before you begin, set your intent that you are asking for your highest good and highest benefit.

Simple clear statements or questions work best. "_____ is in alignment with my highest good," is a clear statement. Statements with "I am" or "I believe I am" also work well.

If you are testing the truth of your self-talk, test one of them. For instance if one of your judgments is that you are lazy, test it. Put yourself in a neutral state as described earlier. Then say "I am in alignment with the phrase 'I am lazy *(or stupid, dumb, not good enough, etc.).*'" You could also say "I believe I am *fill in the blank*."

If you find yourself agreeing with one of your negative judgments, you've found an area that needs to have the trash taken out. When you have accomplished this trash removal in whole or in part, your life will take on greater lightness.

"As we live we collect our past." We can also reset it.

Quantum Curiosity

Be curious in your life. One of the best reasons to get out of bed in the mornings is curiosity about the day ahead. I'm always open to whatever is going to happen. If you stay curious, you can't lose your lust for living. Curiosity is how I became a singer. There is always something new to study and learn, something new to sing. Learning is important to me. Curiosity makes me ask questions. It makes me interested in people, why they make the choices they've made and how they have arrived at the places they're at. How did they meet their spouse, how did they get interested in the job they do?

How people come to be who they are fascinates me. Frequently this leads to new friendships. We can always use an injection of the new to keep us fresh and alive. If we stay in old habits day after day, seeing the same people, eating at the same places and the same food, our lives become stale. For some people that is a comfort, but most of us need this influx of the new to keep us curious and feeling alive.

I never assume that the way I do something is the only way to do it. I try to be open to discovering different methods even if I believe I am already efficient in my practice. Frequently I am taught new, more efficient methods by others that make my tasks easier to accomplish.

I always assumed that when I wrote this book, I would write it in longhand because I like the direct connection of heart and head through my hand onto the paper. Yet, my initial thoughts for this book were dictated into a recorder at the suggestion of a seminar leader. As I dictated, my judges came out to tell me that everything I said was stupid, twee and superficial. I persisted in spite of them and in spite of agreeing with them. As I transcribed my stream of conscious recordings, surprisingly I discovered not everything was horrible and occasional nuggets of gold I hadn't remembered speaking sparkled in the dreck. I didn't let my judgment and fear halt my progress, the garbage can always be thrown out.

I also tried not to worry about the completeness of things. I didn't try to ensure cohesiveness or coherence. The most important task was to get the words out. A half-finished thought can eventually spark a complete thought. Every journey begins with the first step. Don't be daunted by the size of your task, make the first step, do one thing.

Keep looking for the thing you feel you are supposed to do – that you imagine or desire to do. Make the first step in front of you even if it doesn't appear to lead to the thing you imagine.

What Are Your Questions?

...I would like to beg you dear Sir, as well as I can, to have patience with everything unresolved in your heart and to try to love the questions themselves as if they were locked rooms or books written in a very foreign language. Don't search for the answers, which could not be given to you now, because you would not be able to live them. And the point is to live everything. Live the questions now. Perhaps then, someday far in the future, you will gradually, without even noticing it, live your way into the answer.
Rainer Maria Rilke, from "Letters to a Young Poet"

I can live with doubt and uncertainty. I think it's much more interesting to live not knowing than to have answers which might be wrong. Richard Feynman

What makes you ask questions? As a child what were you the most curious about? Did you like to study bugs, sit in trees, color, draw, play games? What piqued your child curiosity?

As you grow older, retaining your innocent child's curiosity serves you well. You can't live in childlike naïveté, but retaining the memory of what piqued your curiosity as a child generates enthusiasm. You can use it to open to the wonder of the world around you in each and every moment. You may not be able to do it all the time, but the ability to retain wonder in your life reminds you of your humanity and your connection with everything around you. It makes your problems seem small and insignificant because you have a place in a great scheme we don't yet understand.

Questions stir things up. Up becomes down or sideways. Everything you think you know can become something else. Being in the energy of the question releases its locks. In your search for answers, you find your way and live your life even if the answers never quite reveal themselves.

Keep asking questions. Wonder at how the world functions or how it can function given all the things we do to mess it up. Open yourself to awe-filled, jaw-dropping wonder looking at the lunar eclipse or a blood red moon hanging so low in the sky that it is practically in your lap.

It's A Relief To Not Have To Know All The Answers

It's a relief to know you don't have to have all the answers and that you're not supposed to have all the answers. How did we ever get that idea anyway?

Mostly answers stop you from asking more questions. Occasionally an answer will trigger more questions, but you must be willing to question whether it is the right answer or the only answer. None of us has a complete and total blueprint for how we are supposed to behave in every moment of our lives and it doesn't matter how long you live or what age you achieve you will always be encountering new experiences. Who has ever experienced old age first hand until you become old? Not one of us will grow older in the same way and it will always be a surprise. In your 20's aging is still theoretical, but when you are 60, you're already there. Surprise! This isn't at all what I thought it would be.

Some aging issues are eternal, but each generation ages differently because of their generational experiences and attitudes, advances in medicine, rapid changes in technology. No one knows what it will be until you get there. You will never have a handle on all the things that can happen along your life trajectory, so give it up! You don't have to know all the answers, you're not expected to know all the answers. More important is to have tools to negotiate the questions.

Having beneficial life skills tools you have developed and used over a lifetime is important. They help you feel capable when you encounter new situations. Whether you want to or not, throughout your life you will encounter the unknown and situations that make you feel uncomfortable.

Not everything makes sense. Sometimes you just have to accept that.

Do the best you can until you know better. Then when you know better, do better. Maya Angelou

What Gets You Out Of Bed?

What gets you out of bed? Is it your curiosity? Is it all the tasks for the day lying in wait? Is it just that it's morning and time to get up? Find something that makes you happy to get out of bed in the morning.

Some people get up because of obligations, getting your kids off to school or getting yourself off to work, joining that long line of commuters. Are you curious to know what the day will bring or do you know that it will bring the same old same old same old? If that is true, and it doesn't excite you, can you inject something into your day to make you excited to be on the planet?

For some that will be trying a new food or restaurant, taking a walk, singing a song, dancing, taking a class. Not every day, of course, has to feel like this, but wouldn't it be wonderful if most days you felt excited about being where you are, even if you are in a job you don't care for, if you know that the job is serving another purpose for you?

Sitting in traffic, take the time to do something that serves you. It's a good time to meditate, a good time to listen to music that makes you happy, a good time to dream a vacation, plan your weekend, do breathing exercises. Any of these can calm you and make you relaxed and happier as you move throughout your day. Set your intention to take a few minutes each day to do something just for you.

Meditation for Quantum Connection

It seems we all agree that training the body through exercise, diet, and relaxation is a good idea, but why don't we think about training our mind? Sakyong Mipham Rinpoche

Why meditate? There's no way I could do that!

I loathe traffic and because I live in LA and have a minimum of 45-50 minutes daily commute *one* way, I spend a good deal of my life in traffic. I listen to books. I listened to the whole of the unabridged-complete-with-author-footnotes version of "Moby Dick" and truly enjoyed it. If the commute is too complicated for literature, I listen to music or something soul soothing. During an especially difficult commute, I might repeat the ho'oponopono prayer just so I can forgive myself for subjecting myself to that mess and to forgive my fellow drivers who just don't seem to see the error of their bad driving ways.

A few minutes of meditation softens my loathing of traffic and opens my heart and my awareness to more of what is going on around me. I feel like it makes me safer on the road because I am more aware and my "spidey" sense encompasses me and extends out beyond my car. Meditation helps me recognize when I am getting agitated so I can quickly return to a more calm self-aware state. If you want to give it a try, I have a free download of the Ho'oponopono prayer with explanation on my website, *BodyInTuneBook.com*.

In the practice of meditation I gather up the fragmented parts of my psyche, and reintegrate them into a whole. I loosen my identification with my problems. As I become more whole, I feel more contentment and fulfillment. This is one of the main benefits and aims of the practice of meditation. It need only take a few minutes. Done daily the benefits accumulate and it becomes easier to detach from your anxiety and worry, to step back and see the big picture. When you see and experience your place in the big picture, your anxiety and stress levels drop.

There are many ways to meditate, apps to help you and hundreds of internet sites. I first began to meditate with a group. Meditating in a group helps because everyone is doing the same thing as you and their energy and attention helps you to stay focused. A side benefit is that you also meet interesting people and make friends.

My very first experience meditating was using a mantra. I received my mantra from a guru and used the repetition of the mantra to focus my attention in the present moment. You can repeat a mantra silently or say it out loud. I still use this method. "Om" is a wonderful mantra for beginners.

You can repeat the phrase "May all beings be well, may all beings be happy, may all beings be free from suffering." Keep drawing your attention back to your heart as you repeat the phrase. I feel my heart begin to open just by reading these words.

I've also meditated using mudras which are hand gestures with symbolic meanings. Mudras make you aware of your own energy and affect the flow of the meditation energy.

Another simple way to begin meditating is to sit comfortably in a chair or on the floor and use an object or picture to focus on. When I first learned this, I used a candle and gazed softly at the flame. A picture or another object works too, but it should be something that frees you, softens you, expands your gaze. That's why a candle works. It's a neutral object. You don't need to do this meditation with a candle or other object, but it helps in the beginning to have something to focus on.

Set a timer at first if you want. Start with five minutes and gradually increase your time. Notice your thoughts and your breathing. When your mind drifts off, and it will, let the thought go and return to the candle and your breathing.

In mindful awareness mediation, your breath is the focal point, and you notice the sensations, thoughts and emotions that arise. When your thoughts drift, you gently bring them back to your breath. When thoughts arise, know that releasing them and returning to your breath is an important part of the practice. Over time it will integrate into each moment of your life.

Mindful awareness is a practice that can be brought into your daily life. As you move through your day, notice your breathing, your thoughts and emotions. When you notice your thoughts are about some future or past event, softly bring them back to the present by following your breath. Each time you do this, you create a moment of peace within your day.

I began meditating more than thirty years ago. For many years, I practiced daily. Even today, I do something each day that feels like meditation to me. When I recognize that I am caught up in stupid, petty annoyances or something difficult, a simple, silent mantra repetition triggers a shift in my brain and loosens the bondage of unnecessary stress and anxiety so I can, again, open to the flow of my life.

Declare Yourself

"We" is a generalization. Generalizations are either boring or wrong and they are a way of hiding yourself. They are a way of hiding in plain sight, even hiding yourself from yourself. If you say "you" when you mean "I," you bury yourself in a sea of others.

When I first learned this, I felt a physical shift in my brain. I realized how much I hid behind the generalizing "you" and "we" when I really needed to take responsibility for myself and say "I." Sounds simple, but don't say "you," when you mean "I."

Declaring yourself can be a difficult thing to do because you must declare your authentic self and to do that, you must know who you really are. That discovery happens over time. Sometimes asking these questions will lead you to a teacher.

Declaring yourself to yourself comes first. Every suggestion offered in this book helps you find who you are and who you want to be in the world authentically. How are you aligned? What is your vertical alignment body, mind and soul? Are you aligned with something greater than you, however you choose to define that? By aligning yourself vertically with a higher spiritual concept, something greater than you, and anchoring yourself into your own earthly authenticity you become who you are and you move through your life with your whole self.

This happens over time and although it may seem to happen all at once, in fact, we are an ever evolving work in progress. By practicing some of the tools I have outlined in this book, you can declare yourself more and more over time and integrate all of you into your whole life all the time. You will stay true to you even when life's most disruptive events seem to conspire against you.

Declare yourself over and over again to yourself. Make your own manifesto of Self. This manifesto is not about demanding anything from anyone else or looking for validation from anything or anyone outside of you, this manifesto is an inside job. Declare to yourself who you are: I AM. I am _____ (a woman, a singer, spiritual, a teacher of the **GYROTONIC**® method, a mother, a friend). Declare "I AM." You could make a list of fifty declarations of "I Am." The first few will probably be superficial but as your list grows longer and longer, the I Ams will become deeper and deeper, closer to the truth of who you truly are.

Fear

We all have fear. Every one of us lives with fear at least some of the time.

There are different types of fear. If you are physically endangered, of course you need to remove yourself from that, but there are other types of fear: fear of moving ahead in your life, fear of doing something you may want to do. Assess the type of fear you are having and if this is something you really want to do, then doing it in smaller steps can alleviate your fear.

The important thing to understand about fear is that it can be a creative force. Feel your fear, acknowledge it and move ahead anyway if the fear is preventing you from doing something you know you really want to do. Whatever you want to do might be too much, too big for you today, but you will change as you move through it and you won't be the same person at the end of your challenge as you were at the beginning.

Making a plan before you do something can alleviate fear. In his book, "Double Your Income Doing What You Love," author Raymond Aaron outlines a goal setting strategy suggested by his colleague, Alan Jacques, that rocked my world and dissolved my procrastination induced guilt. This wonderful method of setting goals uses three levels of accomplishment. His strategy works for any goal but is especially helpful for large, seemingly unattainable goals and unpleasant tasks. It's one of the strategies I used in writing this book (notice the I?).

Simply divide your goal into three parts. The first step is a goal you know you can accomplish without difficulty. This should be a simple, easy step you know you can get yourself to do.

The second level is a medium step, one that is a bit of a stretch beyond what you think you can accomplish.

The third level is what he terms "outrageous." This is the most challenging, the step that is the impossible goal you know you will never accomplish no matter what.

This method sets you up to win every time. If all you can accomplish is the first level and you do it, you are a winner. If you manage the second then you are a bigger winner and, oh my(!) if you manage the third, you've just climbed Mount Everest (in your own mind – but remember mirror neurons!).

For example, instead of looking at a mountain of paper in your office, step one might be to straighten everything into piles. That could be all you do that day, but you have accomplished your task. If you can do more that day, reward yourself, take a break if you want before you move on to step two.

Step two might be to sort through one pile and toss anything that is no longer needed and file anything in that one pile. If it doesn't have a file, put it into the "Outrageous" pile. Step two might need to be subdivided further for all your separate piles, but again, anything you do is counted as a success. If needed, give yourself a small reward for every pile sorted.

Once you have sorted through all of your step two piles of paper, you are only left with one, hopefully smaller, pile, the "Outrageous" pile. Those are the papers that require some sort of attention. Who knows, once you get going with step one, you might feel energized and make it through step two. With that success you could even feel inspired to go all the way through step three! Success builds on success.

No one lives a life completely without fear. This is a fact none of us can escape. We all feel fear, sometimes on a daily basis, sometimes on an hourly basis. The single best way to handle ordinary fear is to be with it and take your time. Look at it, break it down into pieces. Turn around in your mind, face it, feel it, ask it questions, describe it. Describe it out loud into your hand. If it is a color, describe it. If it is a shape, describe it. If it is a feeling, describe it. If you feel it in a place in your body, go to that place and see, feel, touch, listen to it, breathe deeply into that place. Make friends with it. Ask the fear why are you here, why are you in my life, what do you do for me? Listen to how the fear answers. Engage it in a spoken, out loud dialogue. Visit my website, *BodyInTuneBook.com*, for a free download of a breathing technique to try. Write everything down if you need to. Get it out of your body and out of the worn out pathways of your brain so you can develop new neural networks for the quantum being you are.

One of the reasons constellation work is so effective is because it takes what is lodged inside of you, what is stirring and stuck there and puts it outside of you into an energetic field so you can look at it and see what is going on. Getting fear and anxiety out of your body is a relief and automatically lessens it. Constellation work takes what is in your brain and gives it a physical shape and movement.

Write your questions in a journal and listen to the responses that float to the surface. Speak them out loud. What do you do for me? Are you someone in my life? What is your purpose in my life? Begin a dialogue, listen to the answers, validate the responses without imposing any judgment and keep asking questions. That is how to use fear as a creative force in your life.

Bravery isn't the absence of fear. It is the unwillingness to be ruled by it. To feel and know fear and to struggle against your greatest limitations characterize the embrace of passion.

When you get to the other side of fear, beyond the fog, once you are through it, you have more freedom to navigate yourself.

Quantum Change

Because you really don't have all the answers and because you are each day making up each moment as you go along, you must be adaptable to change. The only constant in life is change. It's the only thing you can expect with any certainty. As you meet change you learn you must be flexible. You must accept that your plans will change. You plan and god laughs. You set out with a plan and make goals, but rarely does anyone make it all the way through to the end without having to alter course. When new information comes in, it is necessary to be able to adapt.

People don't behave in the way you expect them to behave. The only control you have is your reaction to their behavior. When working with other people one must discover whether or not you are speaking about the same thing. You may assume that you are defining something the same way as another and then discover you are each defining the topic differently. When working with others don't assume you are each using the same definition of your topic.

Your assumptions can be wrong. You might assume someone is saying something negative about you when that isn't what they meant at all. By ensuring all are on the same page regarding a particular task and each person has clearly defined what is meant by the words they are using, it is easier to find common ground between and among what at first may appear to be disparate points of view to prevent misunderstandings. Conversely, by clearly defining among colleagues their duties regarding a particular task, there is little or no ambiguity about who is responsible for what task.

If I want to check that I understand the intent of what someone has said I will paraphrase their statement and mirror it back by saying "so you're saying _____," listening to ensure I correctly understand what they are saying and not assuming that I understand.

As a trainer and coach I want to provide my clients with an experience that will help them to grow beyond their perceived limits, so when someone says "my ankle hurts," I'll ask them to tell me specifically what they mean by this, where does it hurt, what kind of pain is it, do you feel it anywhere else, so they can tell me exactly where they feel the problem and then I can watch as they do a movement. We can then address the issue together. I might say "I'm hearing you say the pain is here, but is it also going there?"

Bringing clarity into a relationship develops trust which helps barriers drop and communication then becomes more effective. Communication becomes more honest and direct because my client knows and I know that we will work together to define the issue clearly and explore it and resolve it. Don't always assume that you know what the other person is saying. They may be using words that mean one thing to you, and those same words could mean something entirely different to them.

Flexibility vs. Rigidity

Be clear about your goal but be flexible about the
process of achieving it.
Zig Ziglar

Rigidity gets in the way of goal achievement. If you set your standards too high or define your success by a rigid set of standards you are prevented from acknowledging any of your achievements. Because you may never achieve your inflexible definition of success, you always focus on the future when you *will* achieve it, and then you miss out on what's happening today, right now. If you are always focused on attaining your definition of success at some point in the future, you are probably ignoring all opportunities that don't appear to fit into your rigid plan–not only ignoring them, but actually not being aware of them. If you hold on too tightly to a fixed idea, you miss new options.

Holding your goals flexibly and lightly reduces your anxiety over results and enhances your creativity in achieving them. You'll have more fun.

For example, I have a definition of myself as having bad parking karma. So bad, in fact, that someone once gave me a saint card depicting my own personal parking saint! This person seems to have the parking fairies working overtime in her favor, but, in fact, she is more patient and tuned into her intention to find a parking space, alert for clues to an open space. I, on the other hand, am tuned into my rigid anxiety about my bad parking space juju, and often miss open parking spaces right in front of me because I am more focused on my anxiety over not ever being able to locate a parking space instead looking for the signs that a space might be open or soon becoming available.

If you are rigid you keep throwing yourself at an obstacle and bouncing off or possibly breaking up, but if you can flow like water, you can go right around it or over it, even under it. Flowing like water and holding your goals lightly helps you to stay in the moment. When you are present in each moment you are doing what you need to do RIGHT THEN to accomplish that goal. The process is to work day to day, moment to moment, consciously and gently. A seed starts with a single sprout and gently works its way through a crack.

The simple truth: Yesterday has passed and tomorrow is not guaranteed. All you are left with is today. One of my teachers is fond of saying, "Clap three times yesterday and clap three times tomorrow." You can't. Today you can't clap yesterday and tomorrow will be today, so you can't clap tomorrow either.

Knowing when to hold firm and when to flow like water is an art developed over time and through trial and error. Know your goal, but embrace all the seeming mis-directions and mis-steps. There is no way to know in advance what path might lead you to your desired goal. As Byron Katie puts it in her book, "A Thousand Names For Joy," "when you become a lover of what is, the war is over." Don't sweat the small stuff and it's all small stuff.

Pathless

I heard something recently that stopped me ever so briefly and delighted me. I heard someone say that our lives were pathless. Pathless, I thought, thank God! WHAT A RELIEF!

It's saying exactly the opposite of what we have all been programmed to believe and yet, I know it's true. How often you've been told you should follow a career path and a life path and there's a path to success, a path to happiness, a path to health, and then you spend all your time looking for it? And wonder how you've missed it.

You missed it because it's someone else's! It's not yours!

I have thought a lot about fear also and how being on a path might eliminate fear, but it doesn't, does it? A path might be able to push fear off to the sides, but fear still contains and constricts us. You can't eliminate fear. You are surrounded by your own naturally occurring fears and the manufactured kind. Fear is marketed to you. Marketers and power brokers with a vested interest in maintaining the status quo know fear is the best way to manipulate and keep the masses compliant. Marketers exploit your fear to make their sales.

No, the best way to handle fear, your own and the marketed kind, is to face it, know it and walk through it. Fear is a teacher.

A few years ago I spent some time meditating with the Fool card in the Tarot. It's the card with a man ready to step off a cliff. He's carrying a knapsack and a little white dog is nipping at his heels. In my meditations, I placed myself in the card as the various elements. When I was the fool I knew I had to step off the cliff.

The first time I did this, *even in my imagination,* I was terrified of what might happen. I was sure I would hit the ground and die. I had to keep reminding myself that this was only pretend!

Eventually after some time spent arguing with myself and telling myself how silly I was being, it was only pretend, I stepped off. I free fell for a bit and then I began to fly! In subsequent meditations when I stepped off that cliff, I floated on clouds, was caught by angels, flew on the back of an eagle, once I even hit the ground and bounced, but I *never ever died.*

Our lives are pathless. It's a relief to know I can make it up as I go along. That may be terrifying to many, I guess, and yet to some, like me, it is freeing. It also means that to the extent I can, I must be present in each moment so I can make the best choices for me. If I am governed by my fears I cannot be fully present for mc.

I think of all the wonderful creative people I admire. Even though we don't talk about this, somehow they probably know this too. They strike out on their own because they must. Sometimes they feel guided, but what about those dark nights of the soul when the vision gets clouded and fear rises, what gets them through? I can't speak for them, but even in my dark, I feel a bit of light and I know I have to move toward the light. My light is made up of varying mixtures of passion, kindness, curiosity, gratitude, love, nurturing and joy. That light is the antidote to fear and gently lights my pathless way.

Unity In Variety And Variety In Unity

Difference dredges up fear of the unknown in people. But there is unity in variety and variety in unity. Our world is more and more inclusive. We encounter more and more people who don't look like us exactly and who we think don't share our values. Fear of the other, the outsider is part of our reptilian brain, an ingrained survival technique. When faced with the unknown we struggle with this reptilian brain that tells us to fear what we are not familiar with and we must again ask questions. What am I really afraid of? Is it just because they are different, look different? Do I really need to be afraid of this?

At our core, I believe most people want similar things. We want safety of our person. We want the freedom to thrive.

I refuse to believe there is not enough for everyone. I believe we live in a world where, if we are all working for the benefit of ourselves and others, what is good for me must also be good for you and if it is good for you, it must also be good for me. I believe consensus can be achieved if good will is intended. Instead of cutting my pie into smaller pieces to feed more people,

I want to make a bigger pie so that if you have a slice, I can still have my slice. My pie can grow larger infinitely. I don't believe any of us has anything to gain by keeping someone else down. Keeping someone or a group of people oppressed also harms us.

As I write this, in one month, innocent people were mass murdered in Beirut, Paris, Colorado Springs and San Bernardino. And that's in addition to all the murders of innocents that take place around the world daily. I can't understand what drives the perpetrators, but I hold fast to my Knowing that I am a microcosm of the vast macrocosm and that what I think and feel, how I behave towards myself and others has an effect on the whole.

Morrnah Nalamaku Simeona was a Hawaiian Kahuna Lapa'au, a healing priest, recognized by the State of Hawaii as a Living Treasure in 1983. She wrote: "If we can accept that we are the sum total of all past thoughts, emotions, words, deeds and actions and that our present lives and choices are colored or shaded by this memory bank of the past, then we begin to see how a process of correcting or setting aright can change our lives, our families and our society."

She adapted an ancient Hawaiian practice of reconciliation and forgiveness called Ho'oponopono (ho-o-pono-pono). Her work has been spread and adapted by many others since her death, but I use it in the spirit of the Buddhist meditation practice, tonglen. The literal translation of Ho'oponopono is "to put to right; to put in order or shape, correct, revise, adjust, amend, regulate, arrange, rectify, tidy up, make orderly or neat."

The words of the prayer are, "I'm sorry. Please forgive me. Thank you. I love you."

"I'm sorry" means that I am sorry for your pain and I take responsibility for any part I may have played in causing your pain. There doesn't have to be a direct cause and effect. "You" can also mean you. Somewhere and sometime you have done wrong to yourself and others. This is the apology.

"Please forgive me" means I ask forgiveness for any part I have played in causing your pain and suffering. Again, you are not asking forgiveness for anything in particular. You know you need to be forgiven for something. Mean it. And by the way, even perpetrators are suffering. Forgive them in this manner even if you think you had nothing to do with it. Forgive yourself for causing pain and suffering to you.

"Thank you" means I thank you for your suffering on my behalf and I thank you for your forgiveness. Thank you for suffering so I don't have to. Again, mean this with your whole heart.

"I love you" means I love you for your suffering and for suffering on my behalf. I accept you and I have compassion for you.

It's simple and, at first, may appear as a meaningless gesture, but if you practice it with wholehearted humility, it produces a profound catharsis within. You are a microcosm of the macrocosm. You repeat this prayer for your own transformation. You can download the Ho'oponopono prayer with explanation from my website, *BodyInTuneBook.com.*

I repeat this prayer silently many times a day, so often, in fact, that it is practically part of my DNA. It eases my anger and fear in a variety of situations, large and small. I breathe deeply with the words and let the release settle into my body. The more I repeat the prayer the more humble and less judgmental I become. My fear and anger begin to ease and I accept that the offender/sufferer/perpetrator is a part of humanity just as I am and we are in this together. The only way out is together. I choose to do my part to bear witness, to hold space, to balance the energy within myself. I will work with what I know and in that way I contribute to the evolution of the macrocosm.

You Don't Have To Change It All

Here's the wonderful thing about change. You don't have to change everything. You don't have to do everything right. You just have to do enough. If everyone was doing just enough to be their authentic self, to do what they can to keep their corner of the world clean, to be compassionate, it will be enough. You just need to do enough. You don't have to do it all. It doesn't have to be perfect. Change is always toward progression, eventually.

Few among us will ever embrace change with happiness and excitement all the time. Change means disruption, chaos, perhaps the loss of something you hold dear, more work. Change is often unwelcome in our lives and yet it is necessary. Change is the only constant in life and the only thing you can rely on to happen.

A client told me once he had to be certain about everything in his life. He had to have certainty in his life. While I understood why he felt that way, if you can only have certainty in your life then you can only allow the things you know, you can't have any unknown in your life. How do you learn anything new then? Wouldn't that get a little boring? There is no injection of anything new. What do you do when your life erupts, as it almost certainly will at times?

If you have to be certain you can only be certain if you are surrounded by the things you know. Change brings in the unknown. Learning to embrace change allows you to develop a center of your own strength and knowledge of your immeasurable capacities: to know no matter what is being thrown at you or how disruptive your life gets or no matter how many things you love get taken away from you, you are able to connect to your inner knowing and be in alignment with something greater than yourself; that you can handle any wave of change and the stress that comes with it.

Even good change doesn't always come easily but if you can become comfortable embracing change you live in a field of infinite possibility. There will always be heartache, challenges, death and rebirth. It is easier to move through these bumps in the road of life if we don't see them as outliers, but as inevitabilities. They are a part of life, not obstacles in your path, but the path itself. Even chaos sorts itself into order eventually.

Sometimes the path is smooth and at other times it is rough. Acceptance allows space for grace in finding your way through.

The only thing you can change is you. The only person powerful enough to change you is you. The only person powerful enough to stop you is you.

Change may be inevitable, but it can also be your choice.

What is Chaos?

Let us say yes to our presence in chaos – John Cage

Is there anyone who can't come up with a definition of chaos? That feeling of being out of control, of having too many things going on in your life, of having your stability disrupted and the very ground you walk on feel unstable, having all the structure you have put in place disintegrate.

Chaos doesn't even have to be shatteringly disruptive, for some it means being only slightly out of their comfort zone. Chaos can be a pencil out of place on their desk.

Everyone will have times in their life when things erupt, not just one thing, but everything. One thing most of us can handle, but sometimes everything in your life: job, home, health, family, blows up all at once. What do you do to keep yourself from falling apart when everything seems to conspire to break you into little pieces?

This happened to me. I had a period of 3-4 years where everything in my life erupted all at once: home, family, job, career, friendships and health. Like a butterfly encased and preparing to emerge from a chrysalis, my entire world appeared to dissolve completely and I couldn't be sure if any of it would return. I recognized that my life needed to change and I was pretty sure when the pieces reassembled, I'd be ok, but getting through that period required every tool I had at my disposal. I meditated, walked, sang, did therapy, **GYROTONIC**® training, everything I had ever tried that I knew worked for me and I needed them all. Even a simple finger walk through a labyrinth helped. You can visit my website, *BodyInTuneBook.com*, for a free download of the labyrinth I used. I didn't sail through those years, but I was able to maintain my center in the midst of chaos.

Your stability depends on your wholeness within. That's the still point and the place you can go to know you are still you and that no matter what erupts around you, the only thing you can control is your own perception of what is happening and your own response. If you are truly united within yourself mentally, physically and emotionally even sometimes, you can return to stability within chaos. Yes, some things will happen that you feel can't handle. Sometimes stress just seems unremitting, one mess piling on top of another. A practice of daily meditation, whatever that is for you, will get you through: walking, bathing, salt baths, mindfulness. At some point it will end, it will change again. Chaos will sort itself into order. Get help if you need to. Visit friends. Occasionally you need every tool you have.

Acceptance

Finally you have to accept what happens in your life. You have to accept that not everything you want to have happen will come to you in exactly the way you want or think you want. The whole philosophy of always getting what you want can be true but what you want may not always come to you in the way you think you want it or in the order you want it. You can make a plan but you need to accept how the universe brings it to you, how it is offered to you. Your eyes must be open to know that the offer is being made.

You can't shrink from the process of it. You must fully inhabit it. Be honest in assessing yourself and not shirking your duty to take responsibility for your life and to look with as much clarity as you can at your attitudes, perceptions and behavior.

You may need help to develop clarity and honesty, help from someone who encourages you to look deeply and calls you out when you are less than honest. Most of us, left to our own devices, will not truly be honest because it is uncomfortable to see ourselves in a less than perfect light. No one likes to admit their flaws. Have a truth buddy to ensure you are being clear with yourself and not turning away from the things you really don't want to see.

None of us has the perfect life. We have all done things in life we may not be especially proud of, but one fact I have had to learn over and over again is that what I think is not important, what I want to hide and don't want to look at, will trip me up every time. My own culpability in things I don't like about myself must be admitted.

Truly, you are as sick as your secrets. Once those secrets are aired, even if it's just to yourself, the outstretched palm of your hand and/or perhaps one other safe person who will not judge or betray you, the secret can stop ruling you. Make no mistake, your secrets, large and small, do rule you. Whether or not you are aware of it, they govern your decisions and actions.

Inhabit the pain and joy of your process. As someone once said, "The truth will set you free, but it will hurt a lot first."

Quantum Clarity

Be regular and orderly in your life, so that you may be violent and original in your work. - *Gustav Flaubert*

Structure, something that organizes you, is important. Being organized and free of clutter, helps the spaces show through and opens clarity. Isaac Stern said "Music is always what happens between the notes." If the musical notes create the structure, the organization, there is a whole world of space between note A and note B. Note A and Note B allow you to *see* the space and express it.

Structure isn't a prison. It releases time and space. It shows you space and gives you time. If you have difficulty with organization at home, in your brain or time, hire some help to either show you how or do it for you, learn some type of meditation. Being on track and staying on track gives you back your life.

Structure provides you with a home base for your experience and experiments. It can create confidence like the little boy I wrote about earlier, so you can move further out to what you want. If you have a home base it creates stability, then when you go out on a limb, you have a place you can come back to. You can walk out over the edge because you have an anchor if you need it.

Your environment, the place where you live, the things you surround yourself with are a reflection of what is going on within and likewise, your environment can help to create harmony within. If your external environment is harmonious it is much easier to be harmonious inside. Balance is what is needed.

Clarity and Structure

Structure isn't a prison. It's there for you to hold onto at the times you need it, to keep you anchored when you need it, like in times of extreme chaos. Emotional techniques, physical structure you have developed over time, meditation; these evolving structures provide you with a home base of reliability as you move through difficult times. Structure helps to free you from unnecessary chaos.

Organizing your office, home or day, even with an allowance for flexibility in those things, saves you time. If you don't have organization in your office or home, how much time do you waste looking for things? Simple things like creating a habitual place for your car keys or phone or glasses, frees time for other activities, gets you out of the house and on your way with minimal fuss, and most importantly, helps you to be calm and relaxed because you know where those things are when you need them.

An organized base contributes to your comfort and security and provides a foundation for experimentation.

Clarity and Environment

Let's talk about your environment. The environment you live in, your home, the things inside your home, your work place is a reflection of what is going on within. If you don't feel any order within you can help it along by creating some order and beauty in your outside environment. Find a place for you and you alone to create a space where you can feel peaceful and calm. Add some objects (photos, plants) that delight you when you look at them. Organize your yard or your balcony. Put something in it that says beauty to you. Create *Geborgenheit* somewhere in your home.

Clutter affects productivity and performance and peace of mind. The benefits of de-cluttering far outweigh the amount of time spent on it.

Excessive clutter can be a physical stand-in for emotional stagnation and hidden grief. My friend was exceedingly proud of her lovely new home. She bought it on her own and was proud of her decor and furnishing choices and her home was spotless. She also had one bedroom filled with leftover inventory and supplies from a now shuttered home business. For two years, she had been unable to use that room. On one visit I noted she looked different. Her face and energy were lighter, more lively. She explained that she had hired someone to help her de-clutter her junk bedroom. She said, "the cleaning started with a bit of a counselling session and when we started, it was like I was possessed to purge." To her surprise, in the midst of cleaning and sorting she found herself grieving the long ago death of a sibling. Her entire family had repeatedly given assistance to this sibling and had been numbed by the unexpected death and their impotence in preventing it. This external act of cleaning and organizing a very disorganized room somehow connected my friend to her hidden, internal loss and sadness over this death. With this act of cleaning, her frozen emotions began to thaw and she released a burden of grief and guilt long buried inside her.

Environment also means who you spend time with. Be around people who are better than you because they are the ones who show you what you can be. Be around people who are doing the thing you aspire to do. Learn from their skill set as much as you can. You are with the right people if when you check in with yourself, you feel lighter, more energetic.

There are a lot of people who will tell you that you can't. Stick with the ones who tell you that you can. Will they celebrate your triumphs and successes? Will they encourage you when you talk about your new ideas and nag you to get on with them? Do they see more in you than you see yourself? Spend your time with people who inspire you to be the best you can be. In turn, inspire them.

If either of these environments are heavily negative, you are pushing a large boulder up a very steep mountain. If you can, let them go and find new surroundings.

Clarity and Technique

Recently I heard someone say that technique is the way to get to the human part of music. The paradox is that you need to know the boundaries of technique before you can discard or expand them to find the true expression of you. Remember what I wrote earlier about having to start somewhere and you can't start from perfection? There's a learning curve involved. Don't be impatient with technique or in your learning of craft.

It is necessary to begin with a certain amount of structure, to develop a habit of structure and technique. You have to know how to do something and how you do something. That involves learning.

You need to know how to make all the pieces work together–what contributes to making something work. Once there is a structure and framework, you can release yourself to be free because the structure and technique provide a framework, a home base from which you can test boundaries and experiment. If you don't know where the present boundaries are, how can you test them and expand beyond them?

Craft and technique are useful, not to box you in or hamper your expression, but to teach you the overall shape and provide a home base for testing and experimentation. Don't let your boundaries prevent you from exploring. Boundaries help in exploration. Exploration allows you to push your boundaries further and further out.

Developing emotional intelligence, allowing body wisdom are the most human parts of you. The more you truly know about you, the more harmony you will feel within yourself. Disharmony comes from suppressing aspects of yourself that you may not be aware of or that you find undesirable. These aspects, when brought forward and understood, can become your strongest allies.

Benefits Of Clarity

Building a structure and creating organization presents an opportunity for creativity. Without clutter you can see the larger picture and discover places where you can grow beyond your boundaries. Remember what I said about creating space and clarity? Clarity within can be an outside job. If you create an external order it can create an internal *feeling* of order. The outside can give an assist the inside.

It will take some continuous effort. Just organizing once won't be enough. It takes some amount of continuous attention, just like inner maintenance. You have to keep at it, even if it is only a few minutes daily or weekly.

Once you have an external structure pay attention to it. Do the work to keep it in place. Do it at the times it doesn't feel important because these habits are the ones which will help keep your center during times of stress and help you find your still point if/when the world erupts around you. The right amount of structure and organization contributes to serenity. Outside serenity can allow you to open to serenity within. Once there is order you have space to see other possibilities.

Clarity and Confidence

If I set myself a task, be it ever so trifling, I shall see it through. How else shall I have confidence in myself to do the important things? The Richest Man in Babylon, George Samuel Clason

Clarity in thought creates self-confidence and inspires confidence from others. Clarity in thought comes from preparation and knowledge. Knowledge and preparation are enhanced through repetition.

You build confidence by setting and achieving goals – thereby building competence. Without this underlying competence, you don't have confidence: you have shallow over-confidence, with all of the issues, upset and failure that this brings.

Set a small goal and achieve it. Change one small habit and follow through. Use the goal setting technique I discuss in the chapter on *Quantum Curiosity*. Using this technique helps to prevent procrastination by breaking seemingly large tasks into smaller, more achievable ones you can follow through on and finish. Every small step is a win and builds your confidence and makes you feel more competent. Every small step moves you closer to a goal you want to achieve. Wash, rinse, repeat.

Most everything you want is just outside your comfort zone.
Jack Canfield

Take action. If you are scared to try for something and are waiting for the courage, you may never do it. You only gain courage after you do it, not before. Yikes! Start as small as you need to, but take action on something that is a step on the way to achieving what you want. The good news is, the things you do to build your confidence will also build your success.

Focus on solutions. Don't automatically decide you can't do something because you don't have something you think you need. Reframe the discussion with yourself. Ask yourself "what would it take?" "What do I need?" "What would it take to get what I need?" "What kind of help do I need?" "Do I know anyone who can help?" The answers to these questions form your action plan which can then be shaped into smaller, achievable steps.

Don't Let Perfection Be The Enemy Of Good

As I sat in seminars to write this book, I heard lots of people, including myself, say "I am a perfectionist, I can't get it out, I can't speak into the recorder, I can't write, I'm always editing myself." We are paralyzed before we even begin.

When I hear myself speaking that self-talk: "this is crap, I don't have any technique or any structure, I'm not really saying anything, it's all stupid, it's garbage, no one is going to like it, I'm not saying anything new," I say in response (speaking in first person plural to my multiple personalities), "that's alright. Just barf it out. "We'll fix it later or start over." I make myself get it out anyway. In fact, I called the first draft of this book "The Big Barf."

If you want to do anything, you have to make a start. Don't insist on perfection right from the start. Letting yourself be really bad is part of the process of accomplishing something. Insisting on perfection boxes you in and paralyzes you. Insisting on being as bad as you can be flips a switch and allows room for something unconscious and possibly unique to enter into your brain. Try being perfectly bad for a change.

To write this book I must start and follow my initial structure. I can fix it later, mold it into what I hope it will be, but I have to have a starting point and that is my structure. I am not trying to make it perfect even as I am judging my writing and saying I hate it. I will not allow that to stop me and I won't edit my initial impulses. I won't evaluate the content yet. I can't prevent my judges from talking to me—there are too many of them—I just won't allow them to stop me.

OOPS and UBU

One of my teachers, Wesley Balk, wrote several books for the singer actor, developing many techniques to train and enhance singing acting. He taught about the land of OOPS (the One and Only Perfect Sound) and the land of UBU (Ugly But Useful). He wanted his students to explore both lands.

Singers often get stuck and boxed in by insisting on living in an impossible standard of OOPS as the only best way to do something. Our training encourages it, even insists on it. It must be perfect. But the insistence on perfection can hamper our exploration of what is best for us, what is unique about us.

Your desire to be perfect prevents you from even approaching perfection. The perfection desire can prevent you from even approaching good because you are so afraid to not be perfect. My six year old self's decision to be better than anyone else, prevented the adult me from achieving even an acceptable musical phrasing, let alone a good one, because that decision imposed a standard of perfection that was incomprehensible to both of us.

Whose standard of perfection will you use? If you don't allow yourself to explore and occasionally inhabit the land of

UBU, then any standard of perfection you use will remain unexplored, misunderstood or belong to someone else.

If each of us is unique, then why are you trying to measure up to someone else's standard of perfection? Technique is a tool to express your unique beauty. Allowing yourself the freedom to explore in both lands of OOPS and UBU and all the territory in between helps you to achieve the best you can do. Don't let perfection be the enemy of good.

Quantum Failure

Don't Rush Me, I'm Not Done Yet

So if you are young and reading this, and thinking that old age is something that only happens to old people, skip this part. Come back to it when you turn 40 or 50 or 60.

For everyone else:

Age is like art. It's a matter of interpretation. Nancy Pelosi

I worked all my life to become young
no, you can't persuade me to get old
I will die twenty seven.
Jonas Mekas, 2005 unpublished poem (quoted in New York
Times, October 2015)

Mr. Mekas, a 93 year old filmmaker, was interviewed for a *New York Times* article on aging. He believes that detachment from the forces of art and beauty is what causes so many people to get old. "Consciously or unconsciously, I made a choice," he said. "My time is limited, I choose art and beauty, vague as those terms are, against ugliness and horrors in which we live today. I feel my duty not to betray those poets, scientists, saints, singers, troubadours of the past centuries who did everything so that humanity would become more beautiful. I have to continue in my small way their work."

Much research has been done on the diseases of old age, but little is known about why some people age more easily than others, why, indeed, they can flourish in their later years. Nancy Pelosi was 67 when she became Speaker of the House. Mark Twain, Paul Cézanne, Frank Lloyd Wright, Robert Frost and Virginia Woolf are a few of the artists who did their greatest work in their 40s, 50s and 60s.

We are still learning about the biological mechanisms at work inside the brain. New research demonstrates conclusions one might expect and some surprising results.

In a November 30, 2014 *Wall Street Journal* article by Anne Tergesen writes:

... academic studies that date as far back as the 19th century pinpoint midlife as the time when artists and scholars are most prolific. Dean Keith Simonton, a professor of psychology at the University of California, Davis says ... In fields that require accumulated knowledge, creative peaks typically occur later.

Historians and philosophers, for example, "may reach their peak output when they are in their 60s," he says.

David Galenson, a professor at the University of Chicago, analyzed some 300 famous artists, poets and novelists to discover the age at which they produced their most valuable works. He concluded that experimental artists often need decades to reach their full potential. They take years to perfect their style and knowledge of their subjects.

A recent *New York Times* series of articles on aging wrote that people who are more engaged in the world around them are more resilient to the changes that come with age.

Quantum mechanics would suggest that the thoughts and actions of these people are affecting what is going on in their bodies at the cellular level. In the first chapter, I wrote that neurons that fire together wire together. Your thoughts generate electrical impulses which travel from one neuron to another via synapses. You can forge new pathways of synapses at any age. Astrophysicist Brian Koberlein: "Our brain shapes our thoughts and our thoughts shape our brains." With practiced self-awareness you can choose what you will react to and how you will respond and thereby affect the health of your brain cells.

Research suggests a strong engagement with the world around you and your sense of purpose promotes a reserve, an ability to sustain a higher level of damage to your healthy brain connections before they start to break down. The stronger your engagement and purpose the more you add to your reserve.

Your sense of purpose and level of engagement is something you can control. What do you want your life to look like at the end of the day? What do you want your mark to be?

Play Through To The End

Don't give up. I can't tell you how many times I've reinvented myself, how many times I've stopped singing and decided I would never sing again only to begin anew.

Once in a constellation session, I felt myself die. I died to myself and to my idea of who I was. For the next 6 weeks the most I could do was get out of bed and sleep walk through my obligations. I didn't do any singing at all, which previously would have been unthinkable for me. Slowly and gradually over a number of weeks, my desire to sing returned and I began my journey to sing again in an entirely new way. My old self had to die in order for that to happen. Still, many years after, the old me can be triggered and crop up, but now I see that old self as something a bit foreign and I test it to see if it still fits. Usually, it doesn't, and I'm glad for it.

At this point I am singing the best I have ever sung in my life. I have discovered a voice I didn't know I possessed. I may not know where any of this will lead, but I know I will jump through any crack I find. It ain't over 'til it's over. Being a musician has taught me to how to play, not every note is equally important, and I must sing all the way through to the end of the phrase and how I get there is negotiable.

Life is an endless path of lessons in renewal. Growing old may be inevitable, but refusing to fade is a choice.

It Doesn't Have To Be Easy

You have to make the first step, be willing to fail if you want to do something you don't know how to do. A baby doesn't automatically know how to walk. They try to stand and fall and they try again and fall and keep falling until they finally manage to stand. Then they balance themselves and try to take a step, and what happens? They fall! Does a baby ever say to his or herself "I want to walk but I don't know how to do it, so I'm not going to try?" "It looks easy for all the big people around me and it's hard for me, so I'm not ever going to learn how to do this." No. A baby keeps non-judgmentally trying and failing over and over and over again, absorbing the learning from each fall until eventually she/he learns to walk.

It doesn't have to be easy. In fact, it probably won't be easy. Life always knocks you down and you have to keep getting up. Sometimes things go smoothly, and change is constant. There will always be obstacles and difficulties to move through. At times, life is unexpectedly generous and at others, inexplicably mean.

If your perspective is that these changes, obstacles and difficulties are a part of life you won't spend so much time throwing yourself pity parties. The occasional wallow can be fun and useful, but don't spend too much time pity partying, tell the truth and own your own part in the mess, get up and get on with it. Put one foot in front of the other, keep getting out of bed, get help if you need it, go to your job, do what you need to do and look for ways to bring true enjoyment and pleasure back into your life during those periods. The difficult times will eventually come to an end, especially if you help them along by doing what needs to be done.

Embrace Failure

Because ultimately, what's going to matter in your life, the most important gift you have, the most important gift you're given, is the gap between your abilities and your desires. And a lot of people just stop at the edge. They see the gap and they don't try to leap across it. And other fools just—keep going! And sometimes it doesn't work. So it doesn't work. That, a lot of times, is the difference between the real masters and the kind of midrange people. To learn how to work from a position of weakness. Bill Viola

Embrace your failures because they will be your great lessons. One of the important reasons I chose to become a singer is because I knew I was a good musician and had a good voice, but I didn't have a natural technique. I didn't have a talent for how to sing.

Some people are blessed with a natural technical gift or manage to get out of their way enough to learn quickly, but that was not me. Everything I have learned to do technically as a singer, I have had to learn the long, hard way. Nothing has come easily or naturally. I have struggled to learn craft. Struggled because of my own personality quirks (I refuse to call them flaws), struggled because of the physical quirks of my voice and body, and I keep going.

I chose to become a singer because I knew it was the most difficult choice I could make; because I knew I would never be bored. I would always have a challenge to engage me, mind, body and soul. It was the hardest thing I could do. I chose it specifically because I did not have an aptitude for the work. And it still keeps me going. It is my "position of weakness."

Imagine failure. What's the worst that could happen? Then what? Then what? Then what? By the time you finish this exercise, if the worst does happen you have a plan of action in place for failure, a productive, reasonable response. Your anxiety level should drop, you may even be laughing at some of your scenarios. Your weaknesses, reframed, may be your greatest assets.

I Get To Do It Again!

As a student I worked with a famous conductor and director, Boris Goldovsky, who loved working with young singers. We were staging a scene from "Cosi Fan Tutte" and I was nervous to work with him for the first time and had messed up my blocking. Embarrassed and ashamed, I said, "I'm sorry. My fault." Mr. Goldovsky stopped and looked at me. "Don't ever say you're sorry. That is not allowed. You must say, 'Oh good. I made a mistake. I get to do it again.'" His reframe lifted a great burden from me and allowed a revolutionary shift in my perception. Paradoxically, by allowing and not fearing my mistakes, I made fewer of them.

We are prevented from seeing our failures or near successes as important lessons because of our cultural insistence on dualistic thinking: it's this *OR* that, success *OR* failure. Who ever heard of success *AND* failure? Any successful person will tell you that they would not have their successes without their failures. Failures and mistakes can be necessary steps in learning.

Consider: Walt Disney was fired from the Kansas City Star because his editor felt he "lacked imagination and had no good ideas." Oprah Winfrey was fired from her first television job as an anchor in Baltimore for getting "too emotionally invested in her stories." Steven Spielberg was rejected by the University of Southern California School of Cinematic Arts multiple times. Thomas Edison's teachers told him he was "too stupid to learn anything." In one of Fred Astaire's first screen tests, an executive wrote: "Can't sing. Can't act. Slightly balding. Can dance a little." Novelist Stephen King's first book, "Carrie," was rejected 30 times. And on and on …

What do successful people do when they fail? They keep moving forward, showing up over and over again. One hopeful on the latest *Project Runway* television season auditioned 13 times before he was chosen as a contestant and then went on to become a prize winner.

Successful people learn from their mistakes. They are able to discern the difference between what worked and what didn't work. They use and improve on what worked and toss out what didn't work. They don't let their egos get invested in hanging on to stuff that didn't work. Warren Buffett claims letting his ego get the better of him caused him to make the biggest investment error of his life. He learned from that mistake.

Successful people give it their all, but do their best to release expectations. If you have put everything you have into creating something you are proud of, that is the only thing you can control. You can't control the market or people's reaction to what you have done. You can only control yourself. Rejection is part of creating and giving it your all, and knowing you have done your very best is the only control you have.

Don't let failure become a part of your identity. Reframe your failures as early experiments or training. When you fail at something, you're in excellent company. You're in even better company if you learn from your failure, strategize and try again. Change your definition of failure to "learning opportunity" and find a new perspective. Study the failures of other successful people and carry on.

You Are Not Anyone But You

Being a performer is about getting out of your own way. It's what being anything in the arts is about. Get out of your own way and let whatever needs to be expressed be expressed through you. Be the vessel only you can be.

I have sought to explore my limits, but find my limits continually dissolve. One boundary is a doorway to explore another boundary further along. Boundaries, in fact, are markers along the way, encouraging me to seek and explore further.

Technique and craft are important because they provide framework and structure. They provide the initial boundaries. Eventually how all of this gets absorbed into your being and how the framework/craft gets expressed through your own body is up to you. What you feel in your body is up to you, how it works in your body is yours alone. You find it for yourself and it may not be, and probably isn't, quite like how anyone else does it. You are not anyone but you and you can't compare yourself to anyone else, even though we all do and are encouraged by advertisers to do so.

This unique expression isn't limited only to performers. Every person has their own natural expression, mind, body and soul, which is theirs and theirs alone. Failure and success help you define you. Technique and craft help you define you.

The grass isn't always greener and appearances are not always what they seem. How many times have you heard those platitudes, but they are true. Someone may seem to have the perfect life, they may have everything you think you want and yet you may not be aware of the tradeoffs they have made to get that seemingly perfect life. You may not want to make the sacrifices and tradeoffs they made to have that "perfect" life.

Almost all traditional training conspires to pull you away from your own inner knowing. Don't let it.

What Does Success Look Like To You?

Success is lurching from failure to failure without loss of enthusiasm." – Winston Churchill

What does success look like to you? To the real you, aligned with your mission and purpose? Is it a nice house and lots of money, a nice car or is it having a family that loves you, having a job where you are respected and liked and allows you time to do what you need to do or allows you freedom to pursue other activities that are fulfilling? Is it certain qualities you are looking for? If you want the big expensive house, is it really the big expensive house or what the big expensive house represents?

Your current, outer conditions were set in place by the person you were in the past, the person you were then, not the person you're going to be when you get there.

Many years ago I was on a television set playing backgammon with a colleague while we waited to be called to the set. I was killing in the game. I was winning with all my stones on my home board and was ready to bear them off. I began to throw a lot of sixes with the dice and kept exclaiming, "why am I throwing sixes?! I keep throwing sixes! I don't need sixes! Sixes won't help me win this game!"

Throw after throw came up six and finally I had an epiphany as my opponent moved into position to beat me. I was throwing sixes because I was pouring all my energy and passion into asking why I was throwing sixes! I was passionately focused on what I *didn't* want instead of what I needed to win the game. I needed fives and fours.

Immediately, with enthusiasm, I thought "Fives, fives get me off the board, fives help me win the game," and I began to throw fives. With each throw I focused on the number I needed to move my stones off the board and I began to throw a much higher percentage of the numbers I needed and I didn't throw any more sixes.

I did win the game and more importantly that lesson in the power of thought and the creation of success has shaped all my life since. What more concrete example of the importance of my inner dialogue could I get? Anytime my self-talk becomes negative I change to talk that helps me achieve the goal I am seeking. You get what you focus on. What you focus on is what you get back. When you become aware of your own negative thinking ask yourself: "Is it positive? Is it beneficial? Is it relevant?"

What do you *really* want? If you want good for the future you, you set it in motion with your self-talk now.

Quantum Connection

If you are not clear about what you want to do [ask yourself]
who inspires you and hang out with that person. John Gray

Be around people better than you because they are the ones
who show you what you can be. Don't be afraid to learn from
people who are better at something than you are. That is part of
the aspiration, to spend as much time as you can in the company
of people who are already doing what you aspire to do and do it
very well. This will eventually harmonize with you so that you
can also do it very well.

Quantum field theory postulates that there may only be one
electron field. But one or many, at a subatomic level we share
particles with everyone around us. These subatomic particles are
unstable and constantly spin off of their orbits attracted by
another magnetic pull. You spin off your particles to another's
field and they spin off particles into yours. So the company you
keep is very important.

Don't stay in the company of negative people. It doesn't
matter who they are, even if they are your family or your co-

workers, limit your interaction as much as you can, and especially don't make them your friends. Learn protective techniques and use them if you have to spend time in the presence of people who make you feel bad. A regular meditation practice helps you to disengage from negativity.

Most important, spend as much time as you can in the presence of people who are already doing what you are doing and who are better at it than you currently are. Choose wisely. If you want more from your life, you will not learn what you need from people who are at your same level or if you insist on surrounding yourself with negative people or sycophants. You might learn how NOT to do something, but you won't learn how successful people doing what you want to do, accomplish their success.

To grow, you have to be the little fish in the big pond. Never be afraid to be around people better than you because that is how you learn and that is how you can take your place, if you are capable of doing so, and they are the ones who will show you what you can be.

Don't be afraid of failure, don't be afraid of not measuring up. If you have those fears and can't move through them, then perhaps you should be doing something else. That is also an important lesson. Only by putting yourself in your aspirational arena will you ever discover if you belong there. If you don't find that out, you will always be dreaming.

It's wonderful and necessary to have dreams, but if you want them to be your reality, then you must be around people who are doing what you want to do and doing it very well. You may discover that the dream is not the right one for you and then you can adjust accordingly. Choose wisely, and put yourself in good company.

The Wonder Of Being An Artist

Because art is life playing to other rhythms. Muriel Barbery

Is an artist only the person who paints, plays an instrument, cooks or writes? Can anyone see with the eyes and soul of an artist to live a life of artistry and beauty? If you looked at your quantum life with the eyes and soul of an artist, what would it look like?

An artist doesn't worry about knowing every technique in the book and doesn't get bogged down by the "what-ifs." They learn the basics and get to work discovering what else they need to know as they go along.

Making art is a discovery process. Artists know there will always be more to learn and don't let that stop them from making mistakes and learning as they go along. They know one of their best teachers is experience, and as they make mistakes, they know they will discover what they need to know. Artists live in a transient state of being, sifted through the process of creation.

Artists know that if you are making something that makes your heart sing, if you enjoy it, if it connects you to your higher self, then, at the very least, you are an artist in those moments.

Artists don't cultivate a small corner of a huge field and seek to escape to their small corner for their beauty and joy. They are concerned with the entire field of life.

Artists strive to see the bigger picture even in the smallest slice.

Artists lay down their soul, their truth.

Artists are on a quest for discovery and knowledge and clarity and insight into perception, thought, dreams, emotion, habits, mediocrity, and brilliance.

Artists have a need to communicate to and inform an audience, even if the audience is just themselves.

Artists know making art is a habit.

Show a rock to a group of painters and tell them to paint that rock and the result will be as many different paintings as you have painters painting. Artists don't make reality, but a description of reality and truth as they see it. Artists are present in their experience. They live it, flow with it and try to appreciate where it takes them.

Can you live with the eyes and soul of an artist?

Importance Of Coaching

> *Come to the edge.*
> *We might fall.*
> *Come to the edge.*
> *It's too high!*
> *COME TO THE EDGE!*
> *And they came*
> *And he pushed*
> *And they flew.*
> *Christopher Logue*

We have a common saying in English that you have to pull yourself up by your boot straps when you are in times of difficulty. "Just pull yourself up by your bootstraps and get on with it. Forget about it and move on."

There is a lot of truth in that statement but sometimes you just can't do that. Life can throw some serious hard balls and curve balls at you and sometimes you just can't catch them without help. There are times in life when a little coaching can help and there are times in life when a lot of coaching can help. When you are trying to learn something brand new, you may need someone to help you lay out the steps and be your partner in accountability as you move through the needed steps.

You are not excused from doing your own work. The best coaches don't/won't do it for you, they make you do your own work because only by doing your own work can you truly own what you have done and learn truly what you are doing. There is a difference between being coached to move through the steps as you do the work and having someone do your work for you.

If someone does it for you they are disempowering you. They are saying essentially "I don't trust you to be able to do this. I don't have confidence in you." Yet each of us possesses the strength to carry our own destiny, our own fate, to bear our own burdens. At times you may need a little assistance in moving through the obstacles and barriers that get thrown up in the ordinary course of life. That is what coaching does.

I want my clients to have tools to help themselves and honor their own knowing.

I coach in various ways. I coach using the **GYROTONIC**® method and one of my principals in the way I coach is to assist my client to do the work themselves. I give them an assist. I give them hand assists, verbal assists and I help with questions they may need to ask of themselves. In a physical format it is sometimes necessary to give hand assists.

One of the reasons I was attracted to **GYROTONIC**® training is because I could feel how the system helped energy move throughout my entire body. One client described it as "dancing and swimming in the air." Its creator, Juliu Horvath, writes: "I want music in my body and poetry in my body, and I want to be skillful without struggle; it has to come without struggle." This resonates with me because I want that flow in my body too.

Holding patterns in the body restrict energy flow in the body. We become so habituated to these restrictions, we don't even know they exist until they are shown to us and, most often, begin to create pain. By acknowledging the body in all its capacities we can get out of the idea that there is a wrongness to pain in the body. The pain is telling us something, communicating with us and we can dialogue with it. **GYROTONIC**® training assists with movement re-education.

As a musician I was drawn to vocal music because I love the way words interact with music. I love how carefully chosen words and carefully, thoughtfully chosen notes are brought together into alignment within a phrase. In **GYROTONIC**® training, the same thing happens in a movement. The circular spiraling motions have no beginning and no end and within the continuous movement you are in agreement with your body and the movement allows you to find this agreement. **GYROTONIC**® exercises support from without and support from within. The movement patterns assist you to find the support from within that has always been there. It's a restorative and refreshing change from the pounding noise and cookie cutter workout routine. It's fun because unlike other forms of exercise, your payoff is immediate and your body feels good while you are doing it.

What I Do

In addition to **GYROTONIC**® training, I coach singers, actors and other people who may need to do public speaking and anyone who may be uncomfortable speaking in front of others, strangers or otherwise. I have learned useful techniques from wonderful teachers and know they work, because I use them myself.

Wesley Balk developed a metaphor for the war that goes on inside nearly all of us. He called it the lands of OOPS and UBU. The land of OOPS was especially treacherous for singers – the dreaded One and Only Perfect Sound. The land of UBU was likewise undesirable because this was the land of Ugly But Useful and none of us want to go there. He encouraged us (in my case, very much against my will) to explore both lands thoroughly and all of the land in between.

Anyone engaged in public presentation can be trapped in trying to be good, be the best, be perfect, be right and give the best possible performance. Young singers, especially, can be trapped in their attempts to make the one and only perfect sound. In doing so, we put ourselves into a box and inhibit most, if not all, of our natural selves. A free, authentic expression then becomes pretty much impossible.

In rehearsal, if you give yourself permission to explore the really bad stuff, to be really bad and play back and forth between being really bad and your vision of really perfect, you find a middle ground that is natural, where you can relax and think on your feet and stay in the moment and discover new possibilities.

You want to explore as many possibilities as you can because if you are trying to only do the one and only perfect sound or the one and only way to be a perfect speaker or the one and only perfect way to act a particular role, against whom or what are you measuring perfection? Are you measuring against someone else or someone else's performance? If you are, where are you in that? That person may be approaching perfection for themselves, but you are not that person.

Each of us is unique. You can't be another person's standard of perfection. You can only be yours. To find what uniquely belongs to you, what is uniquely yours, what perfection may be for you, you must give yourself permission to explore the full range of good, bad and in between, the full range of possibility, including attempting to imitate your standard measure of perfection, your ideal. Perfection can be perfectly bad and perfectly good. Why not?

Measuring yourself against someone else's standard of perfection or what you think it is, is an impossible task because you are NOT that person. No matter how hard you try you can't be someone else. You can only be you. If you are trying to be someone else, you can't be authentically you. You are not telling the truth in your performance, whether you are singing or speaking or acting, if you are not expressing through your true self. If you are trying to imitate someone else you are not telling the truth. You are not even telling the truth of the character.

Performance Coaching

Exploration of the lands of OOPS and UBU and all the territories in between is an extremely valid rehearsal experiment, revealing and freeing. One way to explore is to measure it. Put OOPS and UBU on opposite ends of a 1-10 scale and move between 1 and 10, between perfection and ugly, with 10 being as perfect as you can make it and 1 being as ugly as you can make it, then try a 6, move to a 7, go back to a 3 and try out all the numbers in between.

Another technique is remove all expression from the text. Remove the capitalization, the punctuation and all stress emphasis and speak the text of the speech, lyrics or lines, in a complete monotone. It seems easy, but try it. You'll be amazed at what comes up. Memorization becomes easier.

Speak your text from vowel to vowel to vowel. Speak your text using only vowels and dropping all the consonants or speak the text using only the consonants. This technique is especially helpful for singers because pitch is sustained on the vowels and speaking only the vowels or saying the entire word but moving from vowel to vowel to vowel clarifies what vowel sound you are actually using and cleans up any extraneous sounds that could be creeping in. It also helps a singer to clarify what modification might be needed for the pitch tied to that vowel sound. For speakers and actors, your diction will become more clear. This also helps to diminish an accent if you are speaking or singing in a foreign language.

Vary the pitch of your speech. Speak high, low and all the points in between. Try different tempi. Speak fast, slow your speech down to painfully slow and fast again, try all the tempi in between those two extremes. Vary the quality of speech. Say your words staccato or link them all together in one very legato, singsong line. When you've tried all three of these approaches, mix them up and/or try all of them at once. The result of all this exploration will be a more relaxed, authentic approach to your speech or song. It will teach you about spontaneity and your part in creativity and re-creativity and being in the moment when you perform or give your speech.

You can experiment with movement while you are speaking or singing. Try physical gestures that make no sense at all in the context of your words. You can make arbitrary gestures with one hand or two, bend your torso, move your legs. If you have a partner to work with, mirror their gestures. Do some research on Delsarte and play with the gestures out of context.

Learning to use energy opens up a world of expression. Performers are taught to project and, in this context, projection always means outward, sending the energy out. What happens if you flip it, receive energy from everything and everyone around you instead of sending it out? Let it expand into your own energetic space. Then from your energy of reception, send a small trickle of energy out. What do you notice? What changes?

What It Offers

Experimenting with all of the foregoing techniques gives you a wonderful freedom and sense of play which carries over into your daily life. You learn how your body truly speaks, what gestures open you and make you feel confident, what your natural speaking pitch is. You may have modeled a particular way of walking or a posture or speech pattern or vocal gestures without even understanding that you were imitating someone else. All the techniques I have discussed: **GYROTONIC®** training (wonderful for discovering how your body moves) and all the different speaking/vocal techniques are ways your own authentic being can be discovered, nurtured and encouraged to emerge. You might discover that some habitual movement or gesture actually makes you uncomfortable or throws you off balance, hampers you in some way and makes you feel rigid. By exploring physical and vocal and facial gestures you expand the range of expression available to you.

There is no substitute for doing the work yourself.

In performing, to get over your nerves, stay in the moment. Stay focused on what it is you need to do to accomplish the task. Ask yourself, "What helps me to accomplish this?" Don't waste time in regret or dissecting something that just happened that may have been less than perfect. Save that for the practice room. You can't step in the same river twice and if you try, you are lost in the past and lost to the present. Let your mistake go and stay focused on what you need to do to succeed in your task. Staying in the moment is what helps you to do it now.

No regrets. Move on.

Gratitude

It is really the truth that the energy you give to being grateful instantly changes whatever situation you're in if you can figure out something to be grateful for, in that moment.
Oprah Winfrey

Gratitude. With so much turmoil happening in the world and all the negativity that surrounds so many of us on a daily and hourly basis, it's easy to forget that we can always find something in our lives for which we can be grateful. With so many things clamoring for our attention, gratitude can get lost as we move from the next thing to the next thing to the next thing.

"Give without remembering and receive without forgetting." Even the smallest kindness should not go unacknowledged. When you give, give freely, without strings, without expectation. A gift with strings attached isn't really a gift.

Take a moment as often as you can to connect to gratitude so it becomes more of a habit. Write it down in a journal, if it helps, speak it out loud or take a moment to acknowledge the thing you are grateful for and feel the energy of gratitude settle into your body. If you repeat this over and over, you cause the neurons responsible for positive emotions to fire and you develop and strengthen a neural network of gratitude which can counter depressive emotions. This leads to a greater connection to the world around you because lack causes energetic contraction, and gratitude encourages expansion.

In gratitude, even for the smallest thing, you create space in all your negativity and through repetition you enlarge that space. In the space of gratitude you see other possibilities, creative solutions for the problems in your life that would not have occurred to you if you were enmeshed only in your pain and lack.

It cultivates an energy of freedom. Repetition of the Ho'oponopono prayer helps to create space for gratitude. If you would like to download a free version of the prayer, visit my website, *BodyInTuneBook.com.*

Thinking deeply about your mission and purpose in life also cultivates gratitude for what you have and encourages contribution of your best self. I believe my mission and purpose is to assist others to transcend self-imposed boundaries and barriers and facilitate a more complete experience of themselves. Your body is a part of your Being and your purpose.

It is invigorating to transcend something that was previously considered an obstacle. It injects energy and purpose and gives you courage to try for more, to ask for more from your life. Remember, you are your biggest obstacle and you are your greatest resource and teacher.

But you are not really doing it alone. At the quantum level you are connected with everyone and everything, and you are resonating with all the others who are on a similar path. Like Roger Bannister and all the other runners, together, in community, you are creating a new morphogenetic field that will make it easier for others to follow.

Do the best you can.

About the Author

Gretchen Johnson is an opera singer, actress, coach and author. In a career spanning more than thirty years, she has performed traditional and contemporary works in a diversity of settings, ranging from Carnegie Hall to a Masonic temple to an abandoned car park to LA's Shrine Auditorium, often in works written specifically for her. Gretchen helps people gain confidence by training their voice, with a special emphasis on the "body" as instrument. Her soul-sharing musical journeys connect people with music, with themselves and with others.

After earning her masters in music from New England Conservatory and stemming from her desire to have a healthy body that could support her voice and her experiences, Gretchen became certified as a trainer in the **GYROTONIC EXPANSION SYSTEM**®. The **GYROTONIC**® method frees the body so that it is strong, flexible and supported. In this way, Gretchen has established herself as an inspirational mentor and uses this system to transform her own and others' lives.

Gretchen's mission is to empower others to believe that, "It is possible to transcend perceived limitations." She is impressively attuned to the needs of her clients and teaches them how to unite compassionately with themselves and others. Using the **GYROTONIC EXPANSION SYSTEM**®, Gretchen's students are enriched and empowered to face professional and personal challenges head on, with a ready body, mind and voice.

Gretchen is a sought-after speaker. "Body In Tune" is her first book focusing on the body as an intelligent and compassionate co-creator in your life and a potent gift for your greater expression and satisfaction.

If you're inspired to transform your body and voice in the art of music-making and life, please contact her at bodyintunela@gmail.com.

www.ingramcontent.com/pod-product-compliance
Lightning Source LLC
Chambersburg PA
CBHW070918270326
41927CB00011B/2619